The
Facelift
Letdown

When Results Don't Meet Expectations
Solutions For Achieving An Optimal Facelift

by

Sam T. Hamra, M.D., F.A.C.S.

Clinical Professor of Plastic Surgery
University of Texas Southwestern Medical School

DISCLAIMER

The information contained in this book represents the opinions of the author on a non-patient-specific basis, and should by no means be construed as the rendering of medical advice nor as a substitute for the advice of a qualified medical professional. The information contained in this book is for general reference and is intended to offer the user general information of interest. The information is not intended to replace or serve as a substitute for any medical or professional consultation or service. Certain content may represent the opinions of the author, Sam T. Hamra, M.D., based on his training, experience, and observation; other physicians may have differing opinions.

All information is provided "as is" and "as available" without warranties of any kind, expressed or implied, including accuracy, timeliness, and completeness. In no instance should a user attempt to diagnose a medical condition or determine appropriate treatment based on the information contained in this book. If you are experiencing any sort of medical problem or are considering cosmetic or reconstructive surgery, you should base any and all decisions only on the advice of your personal physician who has examined you and entered into a physician-patient relationship with you.

This book is designed to provide information of a general nature about cosmetic procedures. The information is provided with the understanding that the author and publisher are not engaged in ren dering any form of medical advice, professional services or recommendations. Any information contained herein should not be considered a substitute for medical advice provided person-to-person and/or in the context of a professional treatment relationship by qualified physician, dentist and/or other appropriate healthcare professional to address your individual medical needs. Your particular facts and circumstances will determine the treatment that is most appropriate to you. Consult your own physician and/or other appropriate healthcare professional on specific medical questions, including matters requiring diagnosis, treatment, therapy or medical attention. Any use of the information contained herein is solely at your own risk. Neither the author, Sam T. Hamra, M.D., nor MDPress, Inc. assumes any liability or responsibility for any claims, actions, nor damages resulting from information provided in the context contained herein.

ISBN: 978-0-9792240-6-5

Copyright © 2009 by Sam Hamra, M.D. All Rights Reserved.

The contents of this book including, but not limited to text, graphics and icons, are copyrighted property of Sam Hamra, M.D. Reproduction, redistribution or modification in any form by any means of the information contained herein for any purpose is strictly prohibited.

No part of this book may be reproduced, stored or introduced into a retrieval system, or transmitted, in any form, or by any means (electronic, mechanical, photocopying, recording, or otherwise), without the prior written permission of both the copyright owner and the publisher of this book.

Printed in the United States of America.

Illustrations by Kathy Grey
Cover Design by T. Henry Litwin
Book Design by MaryRose Graphics

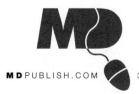

M D PUBLISH.COM   350 Fifth Avenue, Suite 7616   New York, NY 10118

ABOUT THE AUTHOR

Sam T. Hamra, M.D., F.A.C.S., Clinical Professor of Plastic Surgery, University of Texas Southwestern Medical School, is an internationally acclaimed aesthetic surgeon with a career that spans over three decades.

Dr. Hamra attended medical school and completed his internship and general surgery residency at the University of Oklahoma. His residency included a Fellowship at the University of Lausanne in Switzerland. Dr. Hamra completed his formal training with a Plastic Surgery Residency at New York University Medical Center's prestigious Institute of Reconstructive and Plastic Surgery.

Upon entering private practice, Dr. Hamra was introduced to the original SMAS technique, developed by Professor Tord Skoog of Sweden. In 1973, he and his associate, Dr. Mark Lemmon, were the first Americans to adopt this technique. Their award-winning work was published in 1980.

Dr. Hamra was the first to introduce the inclusion of cheek fat (malar fat) to the facelift, which was published as the Deep Plane Facelift in 1990. He was the first to include the orbicularis muscle of the lower eyelid in the Deep Plane Facelift, which became the **Composite Facelift.**

Dr. Hamra is also credited with originating the arcus marginalis release and septal reset. These techniques preserve eyelid fat and use this fat to cover the orbital bone. Today, these operations are performed worldwide.

The Composite Facelift was further modified and refined to its present state several years ago. Dr. Hamra's published description of the *"hollow eye and lateral sweep"* is the first article in medical literature to define these facelift problems and to instruct surgeons on how these problems can be corrected.

Dr. Hamra is in private practice in Dallas, Texas, and specializes in facial rejuvenation surgery, secondary facelift corrections, and rhinoplasty. ❖

PROFESSIONAL AFFILIATIONS

DIPLOMATE, American Board of Surgery

DIPLOMATE, American Board of Plastic Surgery

MEMBER, American Society for Aesthetic Plastic Surgery

MEMBER, American Association of Plastic Surgeons

MEMBER, American Society of Plastic Surgeons

Sam T. Hamra, M.D., F.A.C.S.
9301 North Central Expressway #551
Dallas, Texas 75231-0805
Phone: (866) 773-9181
Fax: (214) 754-9080
Website: www.drhamra.com
Email: drhamra@drhamra.com

DEDICATION

After thirty-five years in the private practice of plastic surgery, I have seen cosmetic surgery develop from what was essentially a simplistic approach to aesthetic procedures to what now is a rapidly advancing specialty, with traditional techniques being refined, and new techniques constantly being created. Finally, people from all walks of life can enjoy a higher quality of life through surgery, which is as logical for maintaining a personal presence with admirable physical attributes, as continuing education is important for maintaining a keen and active mind.

While plastic surgery has a respectable and honorable history, the modern age would not have been possible without twentieth-century pioneers. These surgeons pursued their goals of aesthetic plastic surgery that reflected the results patients have long desired but could not obtain. These surgeons fought conventional bias and institutional blockades until they established aesthetic surgery as an art and a science, respected by the world for great results that have the potential to enhance the lives of people everywhere.

It is to the pioneers in plastic surgery, who taught us all the value of innovation and advancement, that I dedicate this book. ❖❖

ACKNOWLEDGEMENTS

Where does one start when thanking the people who really made this book possible? Since this work is the culmination of an operation that began thirty-five years ago, there has been incredible support from dedicated and compassionate people to whom I am indebted.

First and foremost is my wife Sonia, who has been next to me through every step along the way, and even through the "agony and the ecstasy" that one experiences when dealing with surgical advances.

I have been blessed with the same OR nurse, Ragena Jesperson, for thirty-two years. She knows my thoughts and needs better than I do, and along with Mary Myers and Elaine Jones, who have worked with Ragena, I continue to spend blissful days with help unsurpassed and unequaled. More recently, my surgical assistant Kim Hammond's graceful hands have been there daily for the refinements of my surgery.

My two right arms, Donna Zabojnik and her twin sister Lanna Almand have been in my office for almost twenty-five years and have rendered compassion and organization to our patients and to me. I cannot imagine practicing surgery without them.

My ability to communicate with surgeons through publications depended on two of the most skillful and artistic people I have ever known. Kathy and Scott Grey as a married team are unique, and in fact a dream team, as she is the medical illustrator and he is the high-tech master of photography and computer science with a brilliant grasp of the interface of surgery and technology.

For the past ten years I have had the pleasure of being associated with Dr. Ramsey Choucair, whose surgical skills and impeccable character greatly expanded my life, both personally and professionally.

The superb skill and devotion to patient safety of my anesthesiologist, Dr. Charles Sessions, are absolute necessities when doing surgery that is involved and demanding.

This book came alive with the help of Anne Akers and Wendy Lewis of MDPublish. Their expertise in areas I never knew existed and their honesty and integrity made the delivery of this book possible.

Finally, I wish to thank the many patients who encouraged me to write this book, since it was their opinion that such a book would be invaluable to other patients who could perhaps gain the knowledge necessary to achieve a satisfactory surgical result. ❖

TABLE OF CONTENTS

TABLE OF CONTENTS Continued

*Please Note: Color photos can be found
in the center of the book.*

My Uplifting Life in Facial Surgery

If you have had a facelift and are pleased with the results, there is no need to read this book. I have written it for those who have had a facelift and are disappointed with their final result. It is also for anyone considering a facelift, but who wonders, "what went wrong" after seeing friends and celebrities who have gone through the surgery, yet in time developed an appearance that seems to be so much less attractive than one would expect.

I've spent most of my professional life developing the Composite Facelift, which became complete in 1996. It was for me the realization of what I had worked to create: a facial rejuvenation operation with anatomical changes more youthful than I had seen anywhere before, but without that facelifted look, the "stigma" of surgery. What came as a pleasant surprise to me was that, for patients having a second or even third facelift, this same procedure erased the unwanted signs of prior surgery.

In 1998 I published two articles in *The Journal of Plastic and Reconstructive Surgery.* The first was on new innovations for the Composite Facelift. The second was entitled "Frequent Facelift Sequelae: Hollow Eyes and the Lateral Sweep, Cause and Repair."

The Facelift Letdown

To my knowledge, this is the first article describing the shortcomings of conventional facelifts, and how to correct them. It was not met at first with enthusiasm by every plastic surgeon, but then it was not the first time I received criticism from my peers. New techniques can upset the apple cart in all medical specialties. It brings to mind a saying we had in Oklahoma, "The pioneers get the arrows and the settlers get the land." In fact, after early doubt, many surgeons started to incorporate these new techniques into their practices.

I have found that the patient seeking correction of facelift problems has a much different outlook than the patient seeking facial surgery for the first time. The primary patient looks normal before any surgery is done, has a positive attitude, and is usually delighted with any early result. The secondary patient with an unfortunate and unattractive appearance is usually unhappy, as their goal to have a more youthful face was not achieved. Their results did not meet expectations. After surgery, these patients are even more grateful than the primary facelift patient; the return of beauty after months or years of regret brings a return of self-esteem and confidence.

The encouragement to write this book came from those patients, who tell me that there are so many more people out there who would benefit by knowing that something can be done. I have learned from my teachers, and have shared my knowledge for years with my plastic surgery colleagues though lectures and publications. Now it is time for this information to be available to more patients. First-time patients need to know about possible long-term problems associated with particular procedures. Those who have already had a facelift, and months or years later see unwanted results in the mirror, need to know what can be done to reclaim their beauty and self-confidence.

I am hopeful that this book will be of service both to patients who are disillusioned and disappointed with the facelifts they have had, as well as those who have not had surgery but are contemplating facelift surgery in the future. After reading this book, you will at least know the questions to ask your potential surgeon, whether it is a primary facelift or corrective facelift you desire. There are many well-trained surgeons who do advanced techniques, but you must ask the right questions to determine who has the expertise and desire to deliver the results you want. Even good plastic surgeons too often take normal-looking people and make them look abnormal.

This book should also indirectly benefit surgeons, since a knowledgeable patient is a better patient. Having educated themselves about various techniques, informed patients are better prepared for surgery, and are confident that they are doing the right thing. I also want to shed light on surgery being done by incompetent or untrained individuals who are attempting to cash in on the business of aesthetic surgery.

Finally, I am aware that there are some cosmetic surgeons who will not agree with my approach, and who may even be offended by this book, which is not my intention. All surgeons want great results. Scientifically, it is the technique that surgeons use that determines the outcome, not the surgeon who performs the operation. It is to the patient that we have an obligation to achieve the best result possible. ❖

INTRODUCTION

THE RISE AND FALL OF FACELIFT SURGERY

"My Face Is Not In Sync With My Young Mind"

Plastic surgery is an expansive and exciting surgical specialty. It includes both reconstructive and cosmetic procedures. Reconstructive surgery deals with problems one may have acquired at birth, such as a cleft lip, and those resulting from disease or trauma. Cosmetic surgery, also known as aesthetic surgery, involves the enhancement of appearance. We can then further divide cosmetic procedures into those designed to change ones inherited looks, such as nose, ear, and breast reshaping, and surgery performed for facial rejuvenation.

The primary means for reclaiming a youthful appearance is the facelift. Since the face is the part we present to the world, and aging is something that happens to all of us, I believe facelifts are the single most significant procedure in cosmetic surgery today.

We can also classify cosmetic surgery into procedures associated with the younger patient, and those performed primarily on the older adult. Surgery to change the looks you inherited is generally associated with younger patients. These procedures are well known, and have been accepted for many years. Rhinoplasty (changing the contour of the nose) was developed in Europe in the 1920s and '30s. It has undergone several transformations, with refinements in technique producing results today far superior to those obtained even a few decades ago. Breast reduction surgery has been done for over 100 years, and breast enlargement, despite recent ups and downs in popularity, has become commonplace.

Other procedures generally associated with the younger population are otoplasty (changing the shape of the ears), chin implants, and liposuction. All of these procedures deal with changing the underlying anatomy, and then relying on the youthful skin to shape itself around the new contour of the body.

The philosophy of facelifts is just the opposite. Facelifts are done for an older population, beginning in their late 40s or early 50s. (I do hesitate to use the word "older" for my wonderfully vibrant mature patients! But for the sake of discussion here, it will have to suffice.) Rather than depending on the skin to shrink around new contours, the skin looseness that comes with aging requires removal of skin for facelifts, breast lifts and tummy tucks (abdominoplasties).

Another difference between the young and older patient is that the facelift patient appears to be more selective and applies greater importance to exactly who will be doing their surgery. The young patient today who is looking for liposuction surgery or breast implants seems to know that these are standardized "cookie cutter" operations and is usually content to comparison shop for the best price. The facelift patient, on the other hand, could be characterized as the person who questions their friends when searching for hairdressers, doctors, lawyers, interior designers, or even tailors. They are looking for trusted advice on the best.

Most of the procedures mentioned for the young are shorter in length and therefore less costly—in the surgeon's fees, operating room charges, and for the anesthetist. Fees for facelift surgery are generally much higher, due to the length of the operation and the level of expertise involved. There is also a huge regional difference in fees, compared to other areas of cosmetic surgery. Whereas costs for liposuction or breast augmentation vary little from coast to coast, the facelift surgeon's fees may be ten times greater in some major cities than in smaller ones. The same basic conventional facelift in Manhattan may be three times more expensive than the same operation done 30 minutes away in Long Island or New Jersey.

With advances in healthcare, healthier lifestyles, and better nutrition, we are living much longer today than ever before. In 1900, the average American lived to be 48. Today, the average age is over 78, and even greater in higher socioeconomic groups. The increased interest in facelifts is one of the by-products of our longer life span. As we age and become more learned and more socially sophisticated, it is our faces that can't keep up. As one of my patients told me, "my face is not in sync with my young mind." Additionally, pressures in the professional world have fueled the increase in facelifts. We live in a youth-oriented culture, and both women and men are finding it to their advantage to look younger to successfully compete in the workplace.

Facelifts have been performed as far back as 1913. In some ways, the facelift operation has progressed the least when compared to other tech-niques in aesthetic surgery, such as rhinoplasty and body contouring. In spite of newer names and clever acronyms, many of the most popular facelift techniques embrace the same outdated principle of pulling the face back in one direction, towards the ears. The simplest traditional facelift is a "skin lift," and almost any surgeon, even the untrained, will chance lifting the skin of the face and pulling it back. The magic formula has been known for years among prominent plastic surgeons: a simple procedure plus an easy recovery plus good public relations can produce an impressive cosmetic surgery legend. The success of this formula has been seen for years in Paris, London, Rio de Janeiro, and New York.

I was introduced to the world of facelift surgery when I began my plas-tic surgery residency at the Institute of Reconstructive Plastic Surgery at

New York University in 1970. Having been first trained as a general surgeon in my home state of Oklahoma, I had never had exposure to aesthetic surgery, since plastic surgery was considered to be only reconstructive surgery. Aesthetic surgery was thought to be practiced only in New York, Miami, and Los Angeles — the "glamorous" areas of America. My professors and teachers in New York were in fact the most famous in the world in both reconstructive and cosmetic surgery.

Even though cosmetic or aesthetic surgery was done in larger cities in the 1950s and 1960s, it was basically considered to be a fringe part of the established plastic surgery world. At that time, the plastic surgery societies frowned on cosmetic surgery in general. There was a change in mentality at the beginning of the 1970s, as a number of the most influential American plastic surgeons lent their support and expertise to the formation of an aesthetic surgery society. These men had gained respect by their contributions in reconstructive surgery and had seen the crossover of reconstructive surgery with cosmetic surgery. They were in fact the second generation of American plastic surgeons, but the first generation of true aesthetic surgeons.

The economic boom of the 1970s, led by real estate and oil, provided a very affluent population for the aesthetic surgery market. I had been in practice in Dallas for three years when Betty Ford, the wife of President Gerald Ford, underwent a facelift. I recall well that her photograph was on the front of every magazine and newspaper in America three or four weeks following the procedure. Her appearance was stunningly beautiful. While Betty Ford is given great credit for her contributions to awareness of breast cancer and alcohol abuse, she was very influential in convincing American women of the value of facelift surgery. Beginning at that moment, my surgery schedule was suddenly solidly reserved months in advance for facelifts, even though I was only in my third year of practice. Once thought to be limited to the rich and famous, and done secretly behind closed doors in New York and Paris, rejuvenation surgery was gaining widespread approval. It was like couture became prêt-a-porter. Calvin Klein came into J.C. Penney and facelifts came into Middle America.

With the explosion in popularity of facelifts, consumers have become more and more aware of this operation, but not necessarily for its great results. Many are suspicious of facelift surgery due to some unfortunate and unwanted results.

If facelifts are so good, why do so many who are rich and famous look so bad?

All of the above begs the question from the public, *"If facelifts are so good, why do so many who are rich and famous look so bad?"* Hardly a week goes by in the media without discussion of a celebrity who underwent some type of facelift procedure, and received a result that is neither attractive nor natural. The answer to this question is relatively simple and is the subject of this book. It is not the surgeon who creates or is responsible for unfortunate facelift results, but rather it is the specific technique that produces them. Plastic surgery is no different than any other type of surgery, such as cardiac or gynecologic. A particular type of surgery for particular situations may produce one result, whereas a different procedure would produce a different result. When you travel to cities with a concentration of affluent people, you often observe the very unattractive facial distortions on some of the wealthiest and most glamorous women. Everyone has seen it — it's that pulled-back look and those hollow-looking eyes. Go to a party in Aspen or Palm Beach or any resort area and these ladies look like they're standing in a wind tunnel.

It is ironic that the wealthy have the best jewelry, clothes, and homes, but not necessarily the best facelifts. Obviously these women did not go to incompetent or untrained surgeons. Rather, they went to the "best," and yet the eventual results still appear suboptimal. These poor results are not seen early, but rather they develop over time. The insidious onset of disappointing results may appear six months to one year following the original procedure. These are not complications that can occur following reconstructive surgery or cardiac surgery, where a poor outcome is seen quickly and must be corrected immediately. The early swelling created by surgery of the face will actually hide the true anatomical changes that appear when the swelling subsides and healing is complete.

Having been in practice since 1973, I have had experience with almost every type of facelift procedure. I have made almost every mistake and I have seen almost every complication. For this reason, at this stage in my career, I feel that it is a service to patients to attempt to explain what can happen, why it happens, and what can be done to repair these problems. Facelift letdown certainly is not the fault of the surgeon. Rather, it is the shortcomings of traditional procedures that have been practiced for many years and which have remained by and large unchanged. This is in spite of new and exciting advances, which can produce very attractive and enduring results.

A suboptimal result on the breast or from abdominal cosmetic surgery can easily be covered by clothing.

Facelift surgery is distinctly different from body surgery in its ramifications. A suboptimal result on the breast or from abdominal cosmetic surgery can easily be covered by clothing. On the contrary, facelift surgery is difficult to camouflage. When the result is unattractive, it may generate criticism, ridicule, and embarrassment. The patient is often blamed for the results of the surgery, rather than placing the blame on the technique that was used. I am absolutely certain that unattractive results are never wanted by the surgeon or the patient. Older, simpler, traditional techniques frequently give a pleasant result in spite of their inherent shortcomings. However it is impossible to decide in advance if the technique will result in an attractive appearance for each individual patient, or if that same technique will produce unintended deformities that are hard to correct. ❖

PART ONE

INFORMATION OVERLOAD

Formerly, finding a facelift surgeon
was very secretive
and only passed on from friend to friend.

Navigating Through It All

The process of looking for information about cosmetic surgery has changed dramatically in the past thirty years. Formerly, finding a facelift surgeon was very secretive, with information passed on from friend to friend. Today, magazines, books, television, and the Internet provide ready information about many aspects of having a facelift. It is almost impossible, however, to find information about how to correct facelift problems, which is of course why I wrote this book!

Remember the days when "professionals" such as doctors and lawyers didn't advertise? Those days are obviously long gone. Major changes in the landscape of American medicine occurred in the 1980s, when there was deregulation of industries such as airlines and savings and loans. With that came deregulation of the medical and legal professions, and doctors and lawyers were allowed to advertise. South American and Mexican surgeons had already seen the effect of marketing, which had been allowed in their countries for several years. Plastic surgeons in Brazil and Mexico were pioneers in marketing, as their professional societies did not frown on it as we did in the United States. Many South

American surgeons became world famous by appearing in international magazines and newspapers.

In the U.S., the advent of managed care also dramatically changed the practice of medicine. All surgical specialties were impacted. Decreased professional fees made it seem logical and often necessary to advertise. Additionally, the number of medical graduates had been doubled by the government in the early 1960s. This led to a better patient-to-doctor ratio, but also to greater competition for patients.

The Marketing of Cosmetic Surgery

It has become quite common today for surgeons to retain public relations agencies to promote their names and find opportunities for media exposure. It has been known for years that many of the personalities seen frequently on the society pages of the local newspapers are there courtesy of their publicists. This has now become commonplace in the world of plastic surgery. This is a highly coveted spot for plastic surgeons, since the disciples of the society columns are also potential cosmetic surgery patients. Unfortunately, many of the best-known plastic surgeons have achieved their status by being mentioned in the media, rather than by their surgical accomplishments. Consumers seem to have an ingrained reflex that if they see a doctor's name in print, the doctor must be important. Similarly, if they see a doctor on television, they assume that he must be doing something different, better, or revolutionary to make him worthy of that kind of attention. Regrettably, that is not always the case.

The name of a surgeon appearing repeatedly in a high-profile consumer publication is invaluable. I know—I've been there. But on occasion I have had personal friends in different parts of the country call and ask about a surgeon simply because his name appeared in glossy magazines, even though he had not distinguished himself in our specialty. The presence of his name in that publication was enough to create interest and imply superior expertise.

One must remember that media outlets, such as magazines and news networks, are hungry for stories to bring to their readers or viewers. Flashy new cosmetic procedures with catchy names are great news stories, especially when the feature is brought to them by a publicity agent. Enter the P.R. agents. There may be a company behind a product, a medical center behind a team, or just an individual surgeon who is paying for self-promotion.

While none of this is wrong and all very understandable, there are two problems. In the first place, "new" procedures have not passed the test of time. New does not equal good or better. For example, the "thread lift" is typical of many "miracle operations" that flopped within a year, despite wide press coverage. The results just did not measure up to the hype. Secondly, older procedures like conventional facelifts are emphasized without any discussion of their potential downside or long-term poor results. They have become the accepted "normal and customary" procedures that most surgeons continue to do.

Patient demand drives better and better results in medicine

However, patient demand drives better and better results in medicine. It was a lone group of educated patients many years ago who read about less radical procedures for breast cancer, and then demanded these procedures from their physicians. By the same token, only the well-educated patient will be able to demand and receive better facelift results by learning about advanced procedures.

Popular magazines, daily newspapers, and network television have become the main conduits for information about all aspects of cosmetic surgery. Several years ago, the *New York Times* published an article about the ethical conflict of interest when a surgeon operates on a journalist at no charge or a reduced charge, and the journalist then in turn promotes the surgeon in her publication. This also happens often with books about plastic surgery. Similarly, members of the media often have complementary procedures with lasers, fillers and devices and then promote these products and the doctors who performed the procedures. Among some media this has become common practice.

The perfect combination of a media-savvy surgeon and a good P.R. agent, particularly in major east- and west-coast markets where the media has the biggest presence, can have the desired effect on consumers. Since the perpetual need for information drives magazines and television shows, producers and writers are always eager to be pitched stories of interest and there is a constant competition for breaking a story first.

Although many serious news outlets like *CNN,* the *New York Times, Wall Street Journal* and others, conduct investigative reporting and send writers out to do interviews and to uncover the truth about new techniques, many others accept press releases at face value. Most cosmetic surgeons accept media attention as a good thing, since it creates more public interest and knowledge about cosmetic surgery, which benefits everyone. However, this does tend to benefit surgeons in those large cities like New York and Los Angeles, and helps them create large practices that draw patients from the middle of the country. A surgeon in North Dakota or Missouri would hardly have the same marketing advantage as a surgeon located on the east or west coast, in spite of the fact that he may be better trained and is capable of better results. This guaranteed patient stream may explain why the facelifts offered by the most prominent and well-known surgeons usually fall into the category of conventional, traditional facelift techniques. Some of the more significant and exciting advances in facelift surgery have not been adopted by the busiest surgeons. They simply cannot spend the time to master new techniques and their high-profile clientele prevent them from taking the risk of experimenting with something new. The simple truth is that a limited facelift procedure that an efficient surgeon can do three or more times in a day brings in more income than one comprehensive operation per day.

Beware of Bogus Boards

In cosmetic surgery, unlike many other medical specialties, there is a tendency for surgeons to become well known through articles in the lay media rather than through publishing in peer-reviewed scientific publications. Medical advertising today is pervasive, from magazines and newspapers to websites and billboards. Magazines that report on local happenings in major cities, such as New York Magazine, Los Angeles Magazine, and D Magazine, rely in great part on plastic surgery advertising for their revenue. The problem with advertisements, of course, is that they may possibly be misleading. Consumers are left to navigate through the proliferation of creatively named techniques and to determine the true expertise of the surgeons.

Board certification is considered a minimum standard. It assures you, the patient, that the doctor has graduated from an accredited medical school and, after medical school, completed an approved residency program of at least three years, and passed a certifying exam. Board certification does not guarantee a great surgeon, but it is at least an indication that the surgeon has been appropriately trained for his specialty.

To check on a surgeon's board certification contact the ABMS (American Board of Medical Specialties) at 866-ASK-ABMS or visit www.ABMS.org

While most people know to look for board-certified surgeons, many are still not aware that there are "bogus boards" that masquerade as legitimately recognized boards. California was one of the first states to pass legislation requiring that if a doctor advertises himself as "board-certified," the ad must specify which board he has been certified by. This was initiated to alert the unassuming public to surgeons trying to do cosmetic procedures without certifications recognized by the American Board of Medical Specialties.

Enhanced Photos

For better or for worse, the Internet has become the primary source of medical and healthcare information for many people. Virtually all plastic surgeons today have websites, which allow potential patients to locate surgeons in their area or elsewhere, and investigate those who do specialized surgery. However, you should be careful when viewing websites (or print ads, for that matter) that contain patient "before and after" photographs. Most results in plastic surgery are based on interpreting photos rather than the hard scientific data that internists and cardiologists would consider significant.

While photographs are essential to show the results of surgery, they present several challenges. Digital photos can be easily retouched by anyone with access to Adobe® Photoshop® software. Removal of a distracting background may be deemed acceptable, however, touching up or improving a neckline or waistline is misleading.

Makeup and hair present another problem. It is not uncommon to find photography where the patient is wearing makeup in the "after" photo, but not in the "before." This unfortunate practice occurs in images shown at plastic surgery meetings as well. It may simply be that the patient was unwilling to remove her makeup or put her hair back in the post-op photos, but it can also be quite deceiving. Because of the dramatic difference makeup and hairstyles can make, it may be impossible to tell whether the attractive result was from cosmetics or from the actual surgery itself.

Women have long known that good lighting can make you look younger. Other false photographic representations — deliberate or not — can result from patient position and lighting. For many years, photos showing results of necklifts were frequently helped by positioning patients so they would look younger. A simple tilt of the head can make a big difference in the apparent tone of the neck skin. By the same token, a forehead lift can be simulated by having the patient raise their eyebrows. Lighting can also be used to play up or play down a patient's features. Lighting the patient from the side or above can emphasize shadows and wrinkles, while strong frontal lighting helps hide signs of aging. Diffused lighting can also soften the look of aging skin. Both are common — and often obvious — tricks used when making "after" photographs.

The key with medical photography is to look for consistency in lighting and patient positioning between the before and after photographs. The changes you see should only be brought about by the surgical proce-dure. An occasional mismatched set of photos is not necessarily cause for alarm, because it can happen even in the best of circumstances, es-pecially in the case of long-term follow-up photographs, The camera, lights, and studio may have changed over the years. You should be aware of these subtle patterns of inconsistency to judge photographs correctly. Regrettably, it is impossible to decipher the validity of photos in a magazine ad or web page, since there is no monitoring group to establish criteria for integrity. You have to use your own judgment.

There are some websites that feature patient photos that are not actu-ally the patients of that particular surgeon. Be sure to read the fine print!

Beauty Buzzwords

So-called buzzwords that become part of the marketing vernacular in the lay media can sometimes take on a life of their own. For example, most articles refer to the SMAS, the muscle of the lower part of the face that has been part of the facelift technique since the early 1970s. While patients are now familiar with the word and use it when discussing facelifts, they do not always really understand the meaning of the term and its consequences. Perhaps they have read in an article somewhere to make sure to ask for a "SMAS" lift, or a friend who has had a facelift has offered that advice. Or they have seen a few surgeons who have mentioned this technique to them as being state-of-the-art.

Buzzwords in cosmetic surgery are just that — words that are used to create buzz. SMAS is merely one of the many buzzwords that have trickled down to consumers in searching for the best doctor for cosmetic work or identifying the best procedure to have done.

There is a long list of these terms, some of which mean different things to different surgeons. For example, 'mid facelift,' 'endoscopic browlift,' 'liquid facelift,' 'mini lift,' 'quick lift,' and 'smart lift' are some of the other terms used to describe techniques that have been popularized by consumers and the media.

Anyone can decide to put a memorable name to a technique—whether it is new or old, their own, or an adaptation of something that has been around for years. Relying on a name of a procedure alone can be very misleading. You must truly understand what the procedure involves, and have the proper evaluation of your face or body to find out what you really need to achieve the desired result.

There are many excellent surgeons today who have doubts about whether performing a SMAS procedure is of any benefit at all in facelifting. (Read more about the SMAS in Parts Two and Three.)

Shopping For a Surgeon

Once upon a time, you would go to your family physician, who would refer you to a specialist to care for your particular problem. Rarely did anyone go "shopping" for a doctor. In today's world, savvy consumers shop for their doctors as they shop for their cars, homes, and other major decisions. Americans are sophisticated consumers and most of

Excerpted from MSNBC.com
April 24, 2008

Pursuit of Youth Isn't Always Pretty
By Julia Sommerfeld

"Veda Combs, a 70-year-old plastic surgery veteran from outside Dallas, says it took three facelifts to get it right. The first one, intended to get rid of "that turkey thing hanging from under my chin" left her looking "like he pulled back my face and tied it behind my ears." So she went to another surgeon to try to correct this and at the same time lift up her sagging brow. "This time my forehead was pulled so tight that it looked like my eyes were propped open like an owl. I looked like I was constantly being startled." After reading about Hamra's approach, Combs came to see him in November 2006. Hamra undid the telltale swept-back look with his technique. "Now I look more natural; still, people nearly fall out of their chairs when they hear I'm 70," Combs says.

"You know, when you're all pulled back tight and don't have any wrinkles, it draws even more attention to your age," Combs says. "It's like those older women who try to dress all young and skimpy — it just makes you notice that they're old."

us know that the key is to be educated about all of the options before jumping into anything.

There are clearly many different approaches to facial rejuvenation. Unlike medical specialties where a different approach may simply mean switching a prescription medication or altering the dosage, you have to be very careful in your quest for beauty. New York Magazine ran a feature several years ago where one of their writers went undercover to consult with a select group of cosmetic surgeons, and published the opinions of each surgeon. The span of techniques was unbelievable, and when the article appeared in print, it was surely embarrassing to several of the doctors. The fact is that if a cosmetic surgeon likes a particular operation, he recommends it to most of the patients he sees in practice. Every surgeon has his favorite or preferred techniques that he is comfortable using. These may or may not, however, be the best techniques available.

The flip side is the patient who shops only for one particular procedure without being informed of all the options. Having been raised in the retail business, I fully understand that the customer is always right. But if you go to several surgeons and ask only for a neck lift and lower eyelid surgery, even if that is not the best solution for you, you will probably find many surgeons willing to do it, especially if you wave your credit card. The justification on the part of the surgeon is, "that is what she wanted," even when the results do not meet her expectations.

Of course I can understand why limited procedures are so appealing to patients. Costs and time out of work are the most important factors. Consumers are cautious about signing on for more invasive procedures, unless they have a clear explanation of the advantages over the disadvantages so they can make an informed decision. I also appreciate that younger or less-experienced surgeons may not be in a position to do comprehensive procedures. But prospective patients need to educate themselves to make sure that whatever they have done will not cause regret down the road.

Cosmetic surgery is a business as much as it is a profession, driven by patient desires rather than medical necessity. It is about "wants" rather than "needs." For example, the patient needing a five-vessel heart bypass rarely asks for just three vessels. The OB/Gyn recommending a total abdominal hysterectomy would never offer to remove just one ovary and part of a tube to reduce the fee for the patient. Cosmetic surgery is one of the few medical specialties where the patient actually dictates the terms.

The Famous Guys

I trained in New York with Dr. John Converse, and was surrounded by the most famous plastic surgeons in the world. As our specialty has developed over the past 35 years, I have been close to all of the world-famous surgeons in every country, and see them frequently. We are all friends; we know each other's wives and have visited each other's homes and clinics. We also know each other's techniques well, and have often seen each other operate at meetings. We all attend the same conferences year after year and are well aware of who has changed techniques, and who has really developed something original. There is, as in most professional organizations, the unwritten rule that in spite of conflicts and jealousies, we remain cordial.

When the facelift era began, many surgeons became well known, either as innovators, professors, or as being politically powerful in plastic surgery societies. Many have maintained a presence by organizing yearly surgical meetings and thus maintaining reciprocal relationships from surgeons who present at these meetings. Unfortunately, the young surgeons just starting out sit in the audience hearing the "glamour surgeons" describe the older techniques they do, and forget that the patients of the established surgeons are often happy about knowing who did them, rather than what technique was used. The young surgeon without the big name will never have patients as satisfied with the result if the result does not meet their expectations. Over the last 35 years, the "famous guys" have tended to remain famous until they retire. Relatively few new young bright surgeons have ascended to the hierarchy in recent years. There has been a relative void of imagination and creativity, as new techniques are often discouraged in favor of the old established methods. We have seen much rehashing of the old conventional techniques.

All of the famous guys are really good technical surgeons and are also good people in their own right. Unfortunately, some of the top surgeons have grown so successful that they really do not have the need to do newer procedures. Traditional facelifts can be done quickly, and patients are happy with early results. In a sense, these surgeons are victims of their own success, since they are so busy that there is little time to adopt techniques that have a steep learning curve. Success can inhibit progress, just as discontent can drive one to improve.

Academicians and Spokespersons

Often, when new techniques hit the media, reporters will turn to spokes-people from various medical societies for confirmation. These spokespersons are well prepared to give the official positions of the societies. Because they are speaking for their membership, they are of course cautious about promoting more advanced operations that are not widely used. On the contrary, they may rarely do advanced procedures, and will discuss mainly the basic operations that are considered mainstream in plastic surgery circles.

Information is also often sought from professors who teach at medical schools. Too often, however, academicians are not involved in the day-to-day practice of aesthetic surgery, particularly facelift surgery. While we in plastic surgery depend on these doctors to train young surgeons, that training is (and should be) focused on reconstructive surgery. Spending most of their time teaching young residents to do reconstructive surgery, attending committee meetings, and writing publications leaves little time for academicians to become expert in most cosmetic procedures.

The Power of Television

Since the introduction of ABC's *Extreme Makeover,* over the past few years television networks have promoted plastic surgery with programs that cover every aspect, including actual live surgery. There are even TV programs and websites that specialize in describing horrible results. Every celebrity has been analyzed and dissected as to what part of his or her face or body has undergone surgical manipulation, usually by doctors who have never even seen these celebrities in the flesh.

Extreme Makeover, Nip/Tuck, Dr. 90210, Miami Slice, and many others have been a mixed blessing. Many people saw what could be done with procedures such as abdominoplasty, breast reduction, and other surgeries they never knew existed. These shows introduced the benefits of cosmetic surgery to a whole new group of potential patients. Cosmetic procedures increased 30% during the time *Extreme Makeover* was at its peak, and similar programs have been licensed, syndicated or copied all over the world.

However, the results shown were somewhat misleading, since the reveal presented patients after only six to eight weeks. With new hair extensions, cosmetic veneers on their teeth, glamorous makeup, designer wardrobes, and frequently weight loss, it was difficult to really discern the effects of the plastic surgery they had undergone. It was also never mentioned that the real result of the surgery would be visible only after many months of time had passed, not merely after a few weeks.

With the help of public relations, surgeons promoting new technologies on the nightly news as well as on *Oprah* have become a daily occurrence. Technology led the way in the 90s, when words like "laser," "endoscopic," and "ultrasound" captured the imagination of the consumer seeking out anti-aging therapies. Many of these new technologies have fallen along the way, and in fact some created real complications. Several years ago, after the introduction of the so-called "thread lift" technique, surgeons all over America appeared on television talking about this minimally invasive procedure, where the skin is lifted with several permanently placed barbed sutures. Suddenly, surgeons were seeing many disillusioned patients who had undergone this rather expensive procedure only to find out months later that the effects had totally disappeared, or worse, that had major complications from infections, dents and tissue bunching. Since there is no disciplining agency that regulates this sort of marketing, it is basically a case of "buyer beware." This is very unfortunate, since a bad result can dramatically change the quality of life for someone who just wanted to look better.

Where to Get Referrals

When I get calls from patients in other parts of the country, I normally suggest they ask their own local doctor for names of surgeons held in high regard by their colleagues. It is important to note that while your internist or gynecologist could be the key to finding a reputable and honest surgeon, their knowledge of particular techniques may be only superficial. Armed with the knowledge you will find in this book and elsewhere, it is up to you as the patient to ask the right questions. Ultimately, it is your responsibility.

One significant source of referrals for plastic surgery patients is hairstylists. Hairdressers have seen many procedures from beginning to end, and are the confidants of women who may frequent their salons on a regular basis. I was told at a plastic surgery meeting years ago by one of the older professors that since hairdressers see the incisions in the hair and around the ears, it is in the interest of the surgeon to leave nicer incisions in those places. The problem here is that the incision itself is hardly significant in determining the final result. Some of the worst results I have seen have come from a surgeon who works with a popular hairstylist, who was having surgery done herself gratis as a result of referring many patients.

Many patients are referred to me by their friends. It is not uncommon to operate on one person from a social group and find that this becomes the source of multiple referrals. I remember occasions where the rest of a bridge foursome came after one had surgery. In an ideal surgical practice, the surgeon's reputation and integrity are based on their patient care. Patients refer their friends because they had a positive experience with that doctor. It is the best compliment a surgeon can get.

The difficulty occurs when patients are too quick to judge their outcome. The excellent results they may see during the first few weeks or months after traditional facelift surgery may or may not last. If a patient undergoes a facelift and can be present at social gatherings in the following few weeks or even days, it is normal for that patient to think they have had excellent surgery because their recovery was so brief. It is in this period of time that the patient is so thrilled about their surgery that they will talk openly to their friends, who then assume that the attractive results seen in four to five weeks is the final result. It is not hard to figure that if there was no bruising or swelling, then not much was done. If not much was done, there won't be much of a change.

Most surgeons have in fact felt success after seeing our patients in the early post-operative period. Swelling can actually make the early result look better—it covers up the true anatomical change, which may take up to a year to develop, as the tissues heal. I remember a time when I was just as enthusiastic as the patient in the early weeks, thinking I had achieved a great result, only to discover years later that time was not kind to the anatomical changes I had created. Strangely enough, some patients continued to think the result was wonderful, yet I was person-ally very disappointed. This inspired me to continue making advances in facelift surgery. Unfortunately, satisfying early results have led many prominent surgeons today to continue offering conventional techniques that are easy to do and offer fast recovery. A so-called "mini lift" or "skin lift" may look very glamorous, in the first few weeks particularly, when swelling of the skin creates an almost perfectly lineless complexion that the patient has never seen before.

The more areas added to the facelift, the longer the recovery and the more time it takes to achieve the desired result, but the more complete and youthful the change.

The more areas added to the facelift, the longer the recovery and the more time it takes to achieve the desired result, but *the more complete and youthful the change.* A facelift that can be done in an hour, without the neck lift and brow lift and frequently without the blepharoplasty (eyelids), has become a very marketable procedure. Variations of the so-called "short scar" technique have in fact been done for over 60 years, and yet it has re-emerged today as a very popular surgery. The recovery is easy and, with just a few incisions around the ears, there is minimal pain and often reduced expense.

The general rule is that the younger the patient, the better, as it takes little to achieve an improvement. The older the patient, the less advisable these modified or minimal techniques become, since they can produce a tight cheek area that is out of harmony with the rest of the face, particularly the aging forehead and neck. In time, the stigmata associated with the facelifted look can take over.

Let's look at what happens to the patient who had been so enthusiastic. A year or so later she is embarrassed to discover that the look she thought she had achieved is no longer present. Having referred many friends for the same procedure, she finds it somewhat humbling to seek correction. One must remember that the disappointing results we're talking about never appear early, but develop only after months or years.

My point is that the extra few weeks of recovery after an advanced technique are easily offset by years of a stable result. Isn't three more weeks of recovery a good trade-off for many years of a great look? Even more important is the avoidance of a "facelifted" appearance.

> **As one ages following a facelift, it is not how good you look in time, but how bad you do not look.**

The New Surgeon in Town

Every surgeon has experienced the same feeling when he goes into practice. Having just left the top training program in the country, everyone expects him to know it all. His family is most proud, and there is always a clamor for sending him patients, even complicated ones. Such enthusiasm is normal, as patients from the older local surgeons may be seeing the development of long-term problems with age. But the young surgeons have no bad results…yet. They have not been in practice long enough to acquire long-term results. There is almost a logarithmic explosion in demand for the new "hot hands." I was there as the young newcomer when I first went into practice, and I have witnessed the process repeated many times over the years.

There is an enormous difference between cosmetic surgery and non-cosmetic surgery when considering new surgeons. When a doctor finishes a cardiac surgery or neurosurgery residency, he is no doubt prepared to be at the top of his game, and should be well read as to the most current techniques. If he completed training in the U.S., he will have spent hours in surgery as chief resident, doing the toughest cases, and is prepared to compete with anyone in that specialty the day he completes residency.

Unfortunately, it is not the same with plastic surgery residencies. Great university programs train and prepare great reconstructive surgeons, but give them little exposure to aesthetic surgery. There is not enough time to train these bright residents in both cosmetic surgery and the many facets of reconstructive surgery. Most of them finish with minimal to no exposure to cosmetic surgery. Post-residency fellowships in cosmetic surgery are available, but the time commitment required rarely appeals to young surgeons eager to start practice.

To complicate matters, the young surgeon just entering private practice generally attracts younger patients — those seeking body contouring surgery such as liposuction and breast augmentation. It is easy to become focused on bodywork, and fall into the habit of doing the more minimal facelift procedures.

A facelift practice grows slowly over many years. I have found that it is the surgeons in their 40s and 50s who are doing the advanced techniques. They have already gone through a lot of experience with the more conventional procedures and by then have had some disappointed patients, which drives them to pursue a better result. Paradoxically, it is the older surgeons, who achieved so much success in years past doing what was then thought to be state-of-the-art surgery, who now resist changing. Their time is valuable and newer advanced techniques often carry a steep learning curve.

It is important for you to be extremely knowledgeable and to ask the right questions before having a facelift. You need to be certain that you and your surgeon have the same idea of the endpoint of your surgery. After reading this book, you will understand why disappointments may occur, and how problem areas can be corrected. Do not despair; even a bad facelift result can be made better. ❖

PART TWO

THE EVOLUTION OF THE COMPOSITE FACELIFT

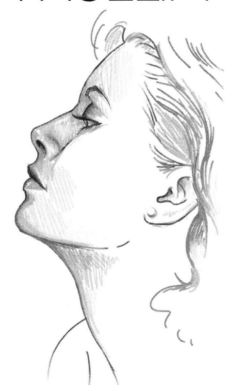

The Composite Facelift
is my contribution to facial harmony

Before we discuss the problems you may encounter in many facelifts, it is important to review your anatomy as it is before anything is done, as well as what I consider the ideal facial rejuvenation goal. In spite of human differences — we are all different, like snowflakes — there is a commonality in aging, and therefore a commonality in the ultimate goals of surgical rejuvenation. After you understand the desired end point of a facelift, at least from my viewpoint, we can discuss in the next chapter the many things that may worry you after you have had a facelift.

The Composite Facelift is my contribution to facial harmony. It represents the culmination of many years of attempting to turn the shortcomings of traditional surgical rejuvenation procedures into better and better techniques. Although other plastic surgeons laid the groundwork with their own fine-tuning of existing procedures, I have had a single purpose in developing this technique: to make sure that you can regain the facial harmony of your youth and retain it long after your surgery. There are many variations to this approach, either from surgeons who have learned my technique or by others who share a similar goal and have developed their own variations. I refer to the Composite Facelift as done by me and countless other surgeons around the world who have adopted this method. It is not a secret operation, as I have published countless articles in the plastic surgery journals, a book *(Composite Rhytidectomy)* and have lectured in most countries of the world where cosmetic surgery is performed. I emphasize that there are other techniques that may work as well, but the goal in facial rejuvenation—truly youthful anatomy— is universally understood and not debatable, and should be your goal regardless of the technique used.

What Is the Composite Facelift?

Traditional or conventional facelifts don't always age well and can result in a "facelifted" appearance.

The Composite Facelift is a next-generation alternative to standard procedures that takes longer to perform and longer to heal, but yields longer-lasting, more natural-looking results. It is based on the concept that the face ages as one dynamic, cohesive unit, rather than as a series of static, independent parts. This means no matter what your surgeon accomplishes with his or her skills and scalpel, your forehead, lower eyelids, cheeks, and jowls will continue their normal predictive descent. Consequently, unlike a reshaped nose that will stay put over time, these elements need to be lifted in unison so when they eventually descend, they do it in harmony.

The Composite Facelift creates that unity by combining various maneuvers into an integrated procedure that surgically changes every part of the face. The forehead and mid-face regions receive the same careful attention (via a brow lift and cheeklift) as the jawline and lower cheeks. More important, the major elements underneath your surface features — the cheek fat (or malar fat) and lower eyelid muscle (orbicularis oculi) — are lifted in tandem with the skin. While previous procedures only repositioned tissue horizontally, the Composite counters the natural descent of the face with a true vertical lift. While I originally lifted the SMAS with the cheek fat and eye muscle, I have concluded that it is best left untouched, as moving it towards the ear actually inhibits upward motion of the cheek fat. More importantly, I believe that the SMAS procedure is the main contributor to the "facelifted" appearance.

As you can see in **Figure 2-1**, the deep structures of the face, the redundant (excess) skin and excess fat of the lower face, the fat of the cheek, and the muscle of the area around the eye all influence the surface topography, and all are moved together to their new positions. It

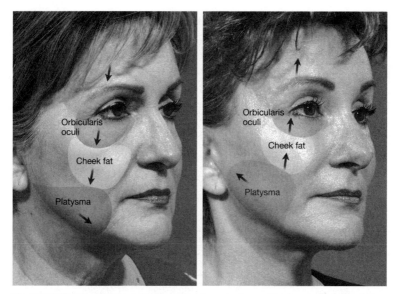

Figure 2-1: Before and after photos show how deep structures of the face age together (left) and how they are repositioned together (right) in the Composite Facelift.

is important to know that the strongest lift direction is upwards, toward the eye. While the cheek fat must be preserved and moved upwards, the excess fat that may be along the jawline giving the "jowl" appearance must be removed. The absolute key to the final result is the ability to move the cheek fat as high as possible and stabilize it there.

It may sound complicated at first glance, but I assure you it is not. The Composite Facelift offers patients a more complete and satisfying facial rejuvenation than the current standard of lifting the lower cheeks and jowls sideways towards the ear, either alone or with an optional lower-eyelid lift. More important, it can correct those stigmata — the windswept pull, hollow eye socket, and bulging pouches along the cheekbone — that may have developed after a traditional facelift.

Let's take a closer look at the evolution of this approach to gain a deeper understanding of its distinct advantages.

How Did the Composite Facelift Evolve?

I began looking for ways to improve conventional facelifts after years of dissatisfaction with their long-term results. The more I saw of the SMAS technique in my early practice, the more I realized that cosmetic surgeons were not always achieving our goal for every patient: to produce a very harmonious facial appearance that's devoid, months or years later, of any distortions or long-term evidence of surgery. In other words, we were able to give men and women a perfectly acceptable initial look but in too many cases it disappointed with the passage of time. To my great satisfaction, the Composite Facelift has reversed that trend. It not only prevents any lasting distortions and remains stable for a long time, but also reverses any unfortunate existing stigmata.

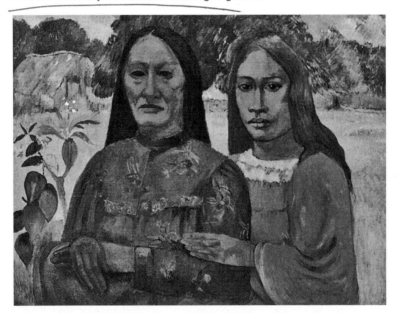

Figure 2-2: *Mother and Daughter,* Paul Gauguin, 1902

Great Artists Showed Us the Way

How did I come to this solution? The old masters offered the first clues. My inspiration for the Composite Facelift actually grew out of observation of the great artists of the past. Through museum visits, I first realized that these men captured, with their brushes and chisels, the very anatomic forces we surgeons seem to have missed in rejuvenating the aging face. Did Gauguin and Rodin understand what was behind every frown line, cheekbone festoon, exaggerated nostril-to-mouth (nasolabial) fold, hollowed cheek and broken jaw-line they depicted so realistically on canvas or in marble and stone? I doubt it.

Gauguin's *Mother and Daughter* **(Figure 2-2)** clearly shows changes to the aging face not present in youth. They didn't know what we know now — that the topical parts of the face fall in a uniform, predictable way, not only retaining a bond with each other but also with the support structures underneath, yet they captured every sign of aging. This means every change on your skin is caused by a corresponding change in the underlying anatomy. Beneath that broken jawline and jowls are sagging facial and neck muscles. With every pair of depressed cheeks and deepened nasolabial folds, there is a loss and descent of mid-face fat.

That widening hollow between your lower eyelid and cheekbone is caused by decreased tone in the orbicularis oculi, the muscle that encircles your eye and helps you blink, squint and close your lids. As it loses tone, its lower aging border forms or deepens a croissant-shaped ridge, what I called the malar crescent, which becomes more prominent over time **(Figure 2-3)**.

The great artists recreated what they saw without such intimate knowledge. Old men were painted with naturally hollow sockets and young people had no jowls and perfect eyelids and cheeks. For many years, plastic surgeons simply accepted a result where the jawline was straightened but the eye socket stayed the same. I concluded that this was a limitation of conventional facelift techniques, and set out to correct it by building on what we've learned about the aging face, gradually filling in the missing pieces. It was the absence of rejuvenation of the eye area that was the driving force behind my quest for a more harmonious comprehensive surgical procedure.

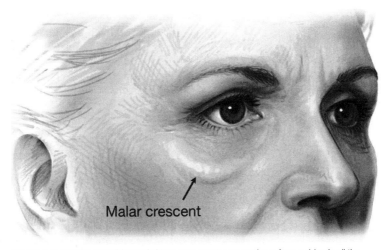

Malar crescent

Figure 2-3: The lower eyelid muscle loses tone as we age, and can form a ridge I call the malar crescent.

Early Years: The SMAS Facelift

I was fortunate to join a pioneering Dallas surgeon, Dr. Mark Lemmon, in 1973. Dr. Lemmon was the first American surgeon to adopt the "Skoog Facelift," the forerunner of the SMAS technique. In 1968, Professor Skoog of Sweden was the first surgeon to lift deeper tissue under the skin. As we learned, the SMAS has been an effective facial rejuvenation tool for decades. It is used every day by the best aesthetic surgeons in the world. For years I was a vocal advocate of this technique without ever doubting its value. As its popularity spread, there was and is still an almost "gang mentality," where a surgeon not doing a SMAS maneuver was not really avant-garde.

In my own practice during the 1970s and 1980s, I had very happy patients return to me years after their first SMAS procedure for a second facelift. Back then I simply used the same technique the second time around. Because the results were what were considered acceptable, it was all that I could do, not knowing that the future would produce bigger and better results. I am delighted now to see patients I operated on years ago, since I can now offer them something much better.

Behind the many satisfied patients who have undergone SMAS facelifts, there are many, many others who can trace the eventual stretches and pulls of an "operated" appearance to a past encounter with this technique. By repositioning the platysma muscle, the SMAS procedure can yield a very good jawline and that coveted initial look. But because surgeons do not always address the cheek fat or mid-face region effectively, it also can eventually lead to hollowness of the eyes and cheeks plus a deepening of the nasolabial folds (nose-to-mouth lines). As mentioned earlier, I have found that better results in both primary and secondary facelifts are obtained by not lifting the SMAS, and have abandoned it entirely.

The Deep Plane Facelift

To address the deepening nasolabial folds, I thought I had found a solution in my first contribution, the Deep Plane Facelift. This procedure, which I developed and named in 1986, and published in 1990, improved the basic contours of the face, and the nostril-to-mouth lines. It went deeper than just the SMAS layers and further than just the neck and lower cheeks. I added the mid-face cheek region to the process, repositioning and tightening the malar (cheek) fat, one of the two anatomic structures key in facial aging. Not only did this soften the nasolabial folds, but it put the mid-face area in harmony with the lower face. By lifting from a level beneath the SMAS layers, this approach provided a thicker flap of tissue with better blood supply, increasing my ability to restore the natural contours of the face.

The deep plane approach proved to be an effective and safe option, especially for the nasolabial folds. I was honored to be asked to demonstrate it in 1990 at live surgery symposia in New York, Miami, and San Francisco. The three host surgeons quickly adopted the operation, and in fact are still using that same exact technique, but calling it by other names. Even with this success, I still felt that it did not give the upper face the same youthful appearance we had accomplished with the lower cheeks. What was missing was that it did not deal any more effectively with the lower eyelid than traditional facelifts.

The Eyes Have It

Since the 1920s, facelift surgeons have used an optional procedure, the blepharoplasty, to refresh the eye area. Most people are satisfied with the upper eyelid portion of this technique because it tends to yield predictably good results. But operating on the lower eyelid is frequently a disappointment, since it can result in a hollow, gaunt appearance over

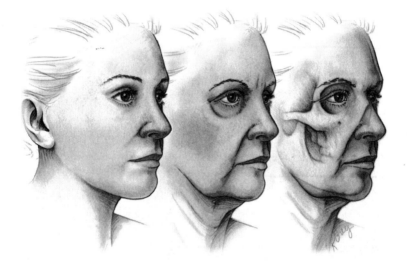

Figure 2-4: Gradual "skeletonization" of the face

time. In a standard blepharoplasty, the surgeon removes the under-eye fat pads and lifts and smoothes the overlying skin and muscle only as far as the orbital rim, the bony ridge along the lower eye socket. The skin can eventually collapse into the depression that is made even deeper by the fat removal.

Since aging creates in all of us a skeletonization of the appearance of the area around the eye, removing the fat simply makes it worse.

Essentially, an "eye socket" is not apparent when we are young, but we all develop it in time as the soft tissues relax and show the outline of the underlying bone **(Figure 2-4)**. This usually starts to appear at about age 40, with the other areas of the face beginning to show the effects of aging soon after.

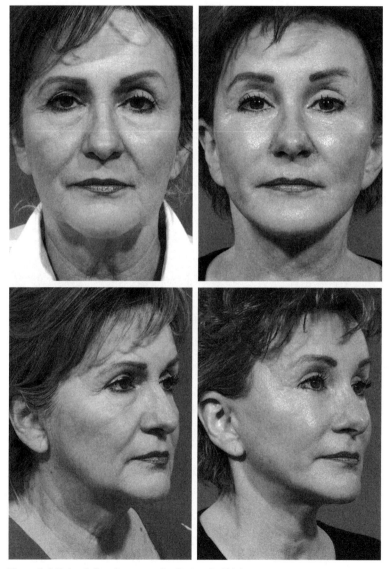

Figure 2-5: Before (left) and one year after Composite (right).

I realized the major role that the eyelid-cheek junction plays in a youthful or aging look. A smooth transition from lower eyelid to cheek is a youthful appearance. Anything else is not. So I considered what it would take to address this essential aspect of facial rejuvenation. The missing elements came together piece-by-piece over many years and became the Composite Lift. It was an evolutionary step, and in a sense, a giant step for me and for the results obtained.

The Endpoint of a Composite Facelift

Since a picture is worth a thousand words, let's analyze the before and after photos of a patient who has undergone a Composite Facelift. The patient seen in **Figure 2-5** represents a typical Composite Facelift result. This lady is an attractive 60 year-old woman who desired a primary facelift procedure.

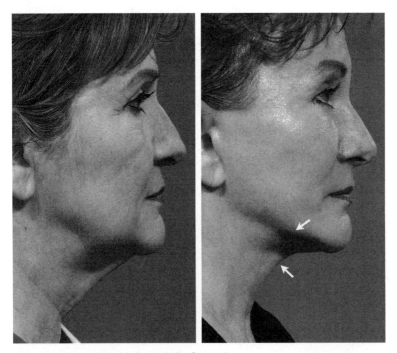

Figure 2-5a: Neck and jowl, before and after Composite

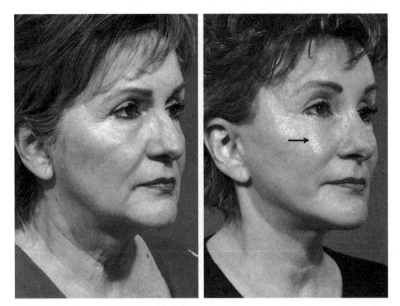

Figure 2-5b: Repositioned cheek mass

Let's look at the normal anatomy and what parts were changed in order to create harmony. From the neck up, you can see dramatic improvement in every area of her face. Extra fat has been removed from her neck and some fat removed from along the jawline, and the "muscle bands" in the middle of the neck have been sutured together. A youthful-contoured neck is the result. Since the neck moves like the knee or the elbow, the skin is loose when it flexes. The neck skin is never as tight as the facial skin even after surgery. The jawline now has a graceful contour. Any extra fat has been reduced. **(Figure 2-5a)**.

The Significant Changes Unique to the Composite Facelift

The "cheek mass" **(Figure 2-5b)** has been repositioned in order to resemble the high cheek mass of youth. *This cannot be achieved by traditional facelift techniques.* The high cheek mass gives a youthful face its beauty. The fat has remained attached to the overlying tissues, which have been repositioned and secured to the bone of the orbit. Its long-

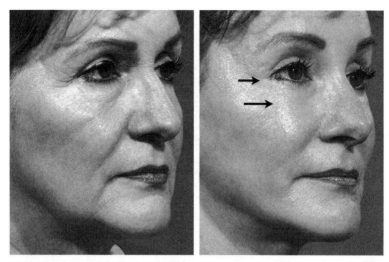

Figure 2-5c: Note the seamless transition created between the lower eyelid and cheek, and the slight upward tilt to the corner of the eye.

term position is assured. I have seen very little change in this new anatomy even ten years after surgery. Attempts to simulate this look with injection of hyaluronic acid gels and fat transfer procedures are at best only fair, and their results are doubtful in the long term. Neither is long lasting. The commercially available injectables only last about six months. and using the patient's own fat requires surgery to harvest fat from the abdomen or thighs every time additional injections are needed. Costs for both are also considerable.

The dividing line between the lower eyelid and cheek has been blended and is now as seamless as it is in a youthful face **(Figure 2-5c)**. This is simply the recreation of the same transition between eyelid and cheek that you had in your younger years. This requires both an upward repositioning of the cheek fat and orbicularis muscle along with a "septal reset," which will be discussed later.

In the Composite Lift, the outer corner of the eye is usually tilted slightly upwards, further reversing the downward movement of the aging lower eyelid. Most patients like the younger look this gives, although this position can be adjusted to suit your personal preference.

The "vertical height" of the lower eyelid is shortened to comply with the contours of young eyelids **(Figure 2-5d)**. This distance, from the pupil to the cheek, must be shortened if you are to see true youthful changes around the eyes. It is a critical component missing from many facelift procedures.

The excess upper eyelid skin has been removed. Removal of this skin may be a once-in-a-lifetime procedure, and is by far the most predictable and longest-lasting part of any facial rejuvenation surgery. This is the key to being able to wear eye shadow — to recreate a crease that serves as a plat-

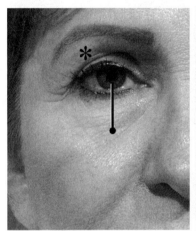 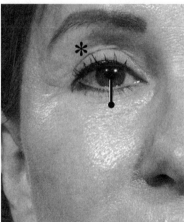

Figure 2-5d: Vertical lines show shortened height of the lower eyelid. Also note the removal of excess upper eyelid skin (asterisk).

form for women to apply their makeup. On occasion, a patient with an inherited deep area under the upper lid may not need to have skin removed.

The forehead has been lifted to be harmonious with the newly positioned mid-face and cheeks **(Figure 2-5e)**. This is the second factor in creating youthful upper eyelids, since a drooping forehead can reduce the impact of an upper blepharoplasty. The frown muscles above the nose have been removed to prevent deep wrinkle lines. The ability to frown is minimized forever. While Botox® injections will accomplish this as well, it requires an injection every three to four months at additional expense.

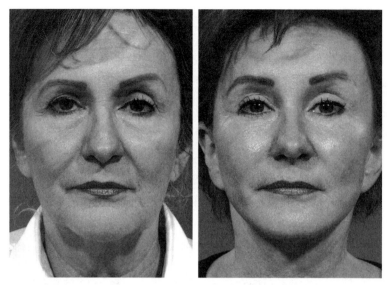

Figure 2-5e: The forehead lift enhances the upper eyelid lift, eliminates frown lines, and can reduce a high forehead.

With the Composite Lift, the surgeon has the choice to make the forehead lift incision at the hairline, which can prevent raising the forehead, or behind the hairline near the top of the head, which will raise the hairline slightly. This patient required a hairline incision in order to lower her high forehead a bit. The loss of hair around a woman's face from

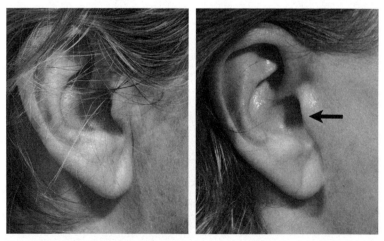

Figure 2-5f: The incision in front of the ear is tucked behind the tragus (arrow), and the incision behind the ear is completely hidden in the hair.

repeated facelifts or certain types of browlifts is a stigma of plastic surgery that is well recognized.

To avoid another one of the telltale signs of facelift surgery, the earlobe must hang at the correct angle and not be pulled forward. The incision in front of her ears is tucked inside the cartilage called the "tragus" and therefore should be hard to see **(Figure 2-5f)**. The incision behind the ear is made high up on the scalp, so a ponytail can be worn without anyone seeing the scar.

Endoscopic forehead lifts, which cannot be done with a Composite Facelift, always raise the hairline.

One of the primary arguments of proponents of the "short scar facelift" is that there is no incision made behind the ear. But since this scar is never seen, I question whether that argument is really valid — the surgeon may just prefer doing a limited procedure.

The best way to observe changes is to view half of the face before surgery next to the same half of the face after surgery **(Figure 2-5g)**. Let's look at the right side of this patient's face to review the endpoints of the Composite Facelift. Then keep these endpoints in mind as you view the photos that follow of primary facelift patients.

Endpoints of the Composite Facelift

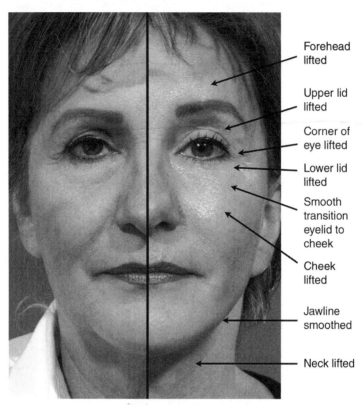

Forehead lifted

Upper lid lifted

Corner of eye lifted

Lower lid lifted

Smooth transition eyelid to cheek

Cheek lifted

Jawline smoothed

Neck lifted

Figure 2-5g: Right side of the face, before and one year after Composite Facelift.

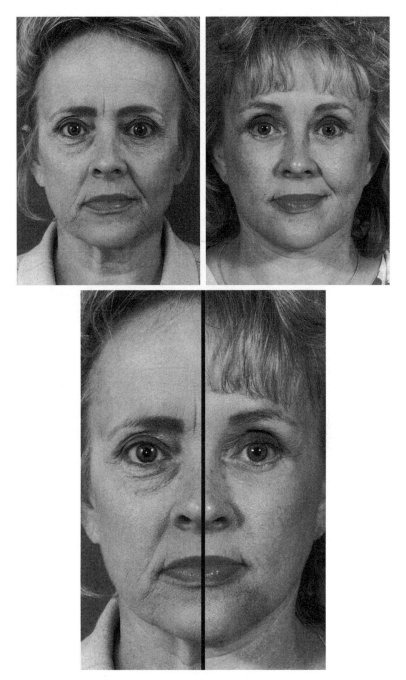

Figure 2-6: Before and one year after Composite. Note higher cheek mass and smooth under-eye contour.

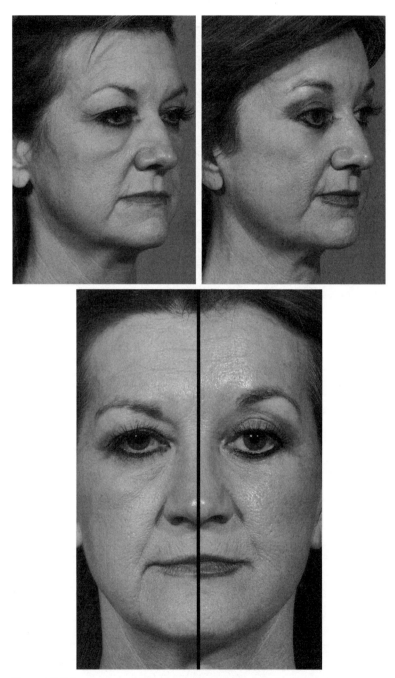

Figure 2-7: Before and one year after Composite Facelift. Note elimination of malar crescent.

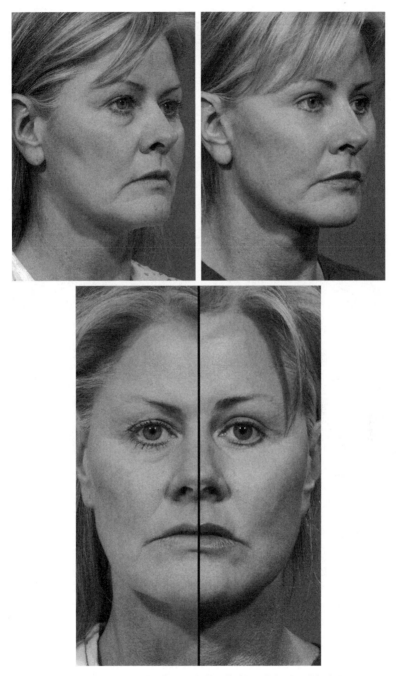

Figure 2-8: Before and one year after Composite Facelift. Note elimination of the hollow eye.

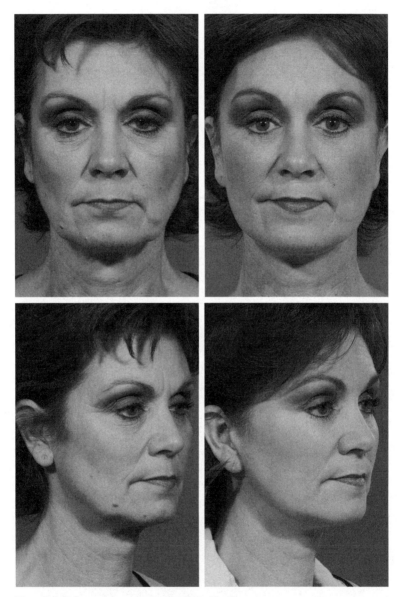

Figure 2-9: Before and one year after Composite Facelift.

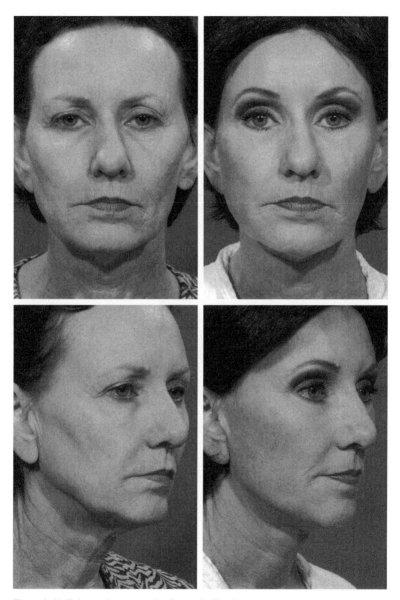

Figure 2-10: Before and one year after Composite Facelift.

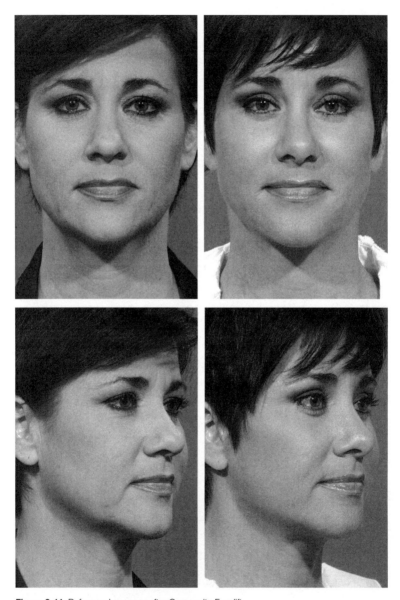

Figure 2-11: Before and one year after Composite Facelift.

How Does The Composite Facelift Work?

The Composite Facelift offers patients a youthful, harmonious contour of the face by preserving the relationship between the skin and the deep anatomical structures most responsible for the signs of aging. It incorporates various surgical maneuvers into a single operation that goes deep and wide to produce the most natural, long-term outcome, whether it is your first facial surgery or a corrective procedure.

Like the deep plane technique, the Composite elevates both the *redundant skin of the lower face and mid-face cheek fat.* Of the two,

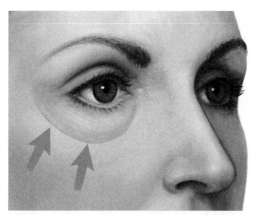

Figure 2-12a: The eyelid muscle is repositioned above the ridge at the edge of the eye socket.

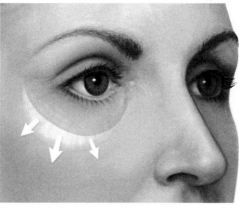

Figure 2-12b: The under-eye fat is extended down over the ridge to soften the transition between eyelid and cheek.

the mid-face cheek fat is by the most important. Its elevation to its original youthful position is responsible for the youthful-looking high cheek mass. The platysma muscle is of much less importance with a Composite Facelift, as lifting the SMAS (which includes the platysma) is not necessary to achieve impressive results.

The Composite also deals effectively with the lower eyelid/upper cheek area, a portion of the face that had been overlooked for years.

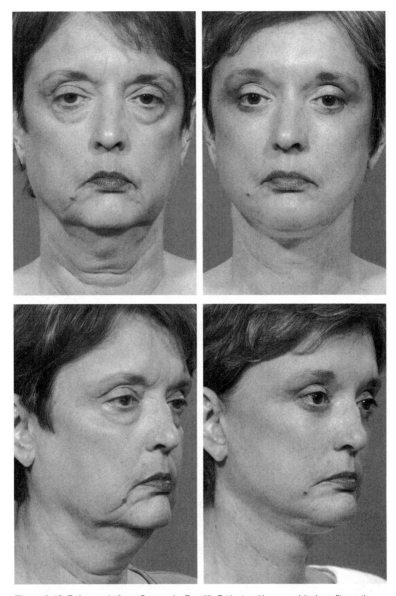

Figure 2-13: Before and after a Composite Facelift. Patients with an overbite benefit greatly from the addition of a chin implant.

When I added the eyelid muscle to the facelift "flap" in 1990, I converted the Deep Plane Facelift to a new technique, which I christened the Composite Facelift. Besides making the blepharoplasty an integral part of the facelift, the Composite technique goes one step further. In 1992, I was the first to preserve all of the eyelid fat and move it over the orbital bone. I published the procedure in 1995. This approach worked well, but I took it a step further by incorporating an even more advanced lower eyelid fat manipulation, the septal reset.

I developed the septal reset to soften the transition between the lower eyelid and the cheekbone. This is the most important step in recreating a youthful eyelid-cheek junction. After moving the orbicularis muscle to its original youthful position above the orbital bone **(Figure 2-12a)**, I reposition the orbital fat with its covering (called the orbital septum) down over the edge of the eye socket on top of the cheek bone **(Figure 2-12b)**. Moving these tissues beyond the rim of the bone,

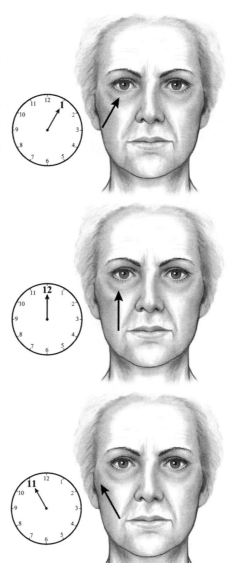

Figure 2-14: Directions of lift

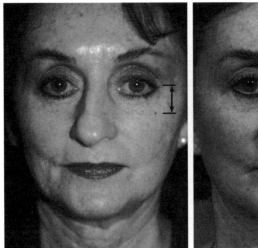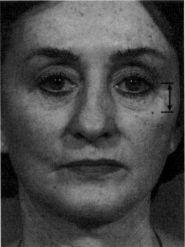

Figure 2-15a: Before and after conventional facelift. No change in the "vertical height" of the lower lid.

rather than just to it, was key in creating a smoother eye contour than we had been able to achieve with other techniques. In fact, maneuvering various facial structures vertically distinguishes this approach even further from previous techniques, including the Deep Plane Facelift.

Figure 2-13 shows an excellent example of where the eyelid-cheek junction is totally obliterated and becomes seamless. The cheek fat has been elevated to a high youthful position and the lower face and neck have been improved with fat removal and the addition of a chin implant. (See her color photographs to appreciate the movement of the fat.)

The best way to understand the difference in facelift directions of lift, or vectors, is shown in the drawing of these three faces **(Figure 2-14)** as they relate to a clock. The Composite Facelift's major direction of lift is approximately 1:00, meaning the facial tissues are moved and fixed in a "superior medial" direction. Other vertical vector techniques such as the subperiosteal cheeklift are almost a 12:00 vector, and can be very effective. All conventional facelifts such as skin lifts, SMAS lifts, and deep plane lifts move the tissues in a "superior lateral" vector, or at 11:00 on

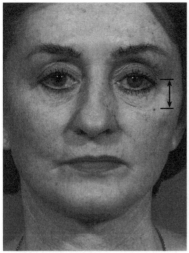
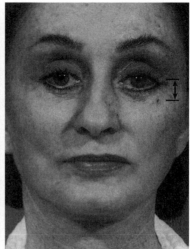

Figure 2-15b: Before and after Composite Facelift.

the clock. Some work well, but always without the ability to effectively rejuvenate the lower eyelid area, which I consider a real disadvantage.

You can easily observe the difference between a conventional facelift and a Composite Facelift when the same patient has had both procedures. Even though this patient received a pleasant

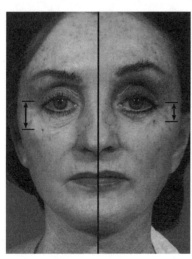

Figure 2-15c: Left: after conventional facelift and before Composite. Right: After Composite Facelift.

change with her first facelift, a conventional procedure **(Figure 2-15a)**, the arrows show how the vertical height of her orbit did not change.

Her original surgeon is a friend of mine and referred her to me, as she wanted a more complete look and he does not do this operation. After the Composite Lift **(Figure 2-15b)**, the cheek mass is higher, the lower eyelid is convex rather than concave, and the brow position matches the new face. You can see that the mole on her cheek has moved in the *superio-medial* direction (up and to the middle). The half-and-half photo **(Figure 2-15c)** gives an accurate comparison between the same side before and after the Composite Facelift.

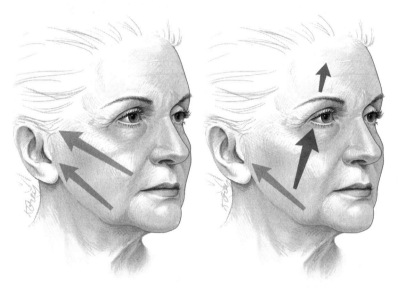

Figure 2-16: Arrows show direction of lift: only toward the ear in conventional facelifts, but the Composite adds a strong vertical vector.

The Essential Differences and Advantages

The easiest way to understand the major differences between the conventional facelift and the Composite Facelift is with arrows representing the vectors (directions) of the two techniques **(Figure 2-16)**.

With the Composite technique, we are able to balance and counter every horizontal pull, particularly of the lower face, with a vertical lift, which also counters the natural descent of the face. By also elevating the forehead, this approach ensures that the soft tissues of your face are draped from the highest possible point to guarantee the smoothest possible look. Because of this, the upper parts of the face will never come crashing down over the operated lower parts of the face. This harmony is maintained for years.

Patients often say, "Doctor, can't you just put
a twist on the top of my head?" That is pretty much
what the Composite Facelift does!

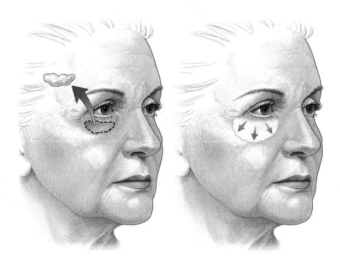

Figure 2-17: Fat removal can contribute to an aged appearance. Repositioning the fat can restore the smooth contour of youth.

The easiest way to understand the difference between the traditional blepharoplasty and the septal reset is shown in **Figure 2-17**. Traditionally, eyelid fat is usually taken out. With the septal reset, the fat and its thin but strong cover, the septum orbitale, is sewn down over the rim of the orbital bone.

If you want to remember the most important different between conventional procedures and the Composite Facelift, these diagrams essentially tell the whole story.

The Composite restores the youthful elegance of the face by overcoming the many limitations of traditional procedures. By bundling a variety of maneuvers into a single operation, surgeons can totally rejuvenate your cheeks, forehead, and eyelids. They are no longer limited by the segmented approach of a conventional or SMAS procedure, and can take on those parts of the face that were traditionally too difficult to treat. For instance, by lifting the cheek fat **(Figure 2-18)** that naturally descends in the mid-face region, we can improve the nasolabial folds.

Because this surgery keeps adjacent areas together, lifts in multiple directions, and preserves the lower eyelid muscle and fat, the surgeon can

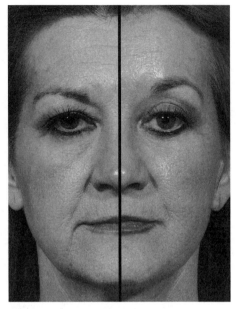

Figure 2-18: Comparing the right side of the face, before and after Composite. As the cheek fat is lifted, the nasolabial fold (the line from the side of the nose to the mouth) is softened and the "malar crescent" problem is corrected.

do more than just promise a lasting youthful contour. And those telltale distortions are nearly a thing of the past…

The End of Lateral Sweep

By offsetting every horizontal lift toward the ears with a vertical lift (or more correctly "superior-medial" lift) toward the eyes, the Composite procedure reverses the face's natural gravitational fall. Your aging lower eyelids and cheeks are returned to their original youthful position **(Figure 2-19)**. Lifting the skin and underlying muscle and fat in this direction also helps prevent the most common distortion of a standard facelift, which is known as the "lateral sweep." This is the stretching of the lower face that often surfaces after a standard facelift. Not all conventional or SMAS facelifts end up with a lateral sweep, but all of them have the potential to

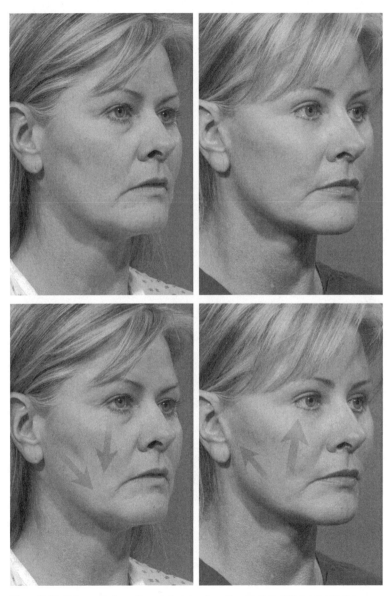

Figure 2-19: Before and after a Composite procedure. The direction of lift is opposite the direction of "fall."

develop this "pulled" look. This is because the tight jawline created by repositioning the SMAS horizontally is stronger and lasts longer than the horizontal repositioning of the tissues of the cheek. The cheek skin and fat can relax in time **(Figure 2-20)**, while the jawline remains taut. When this happens, the difference in tensions reveals itself as the lateral sweep.

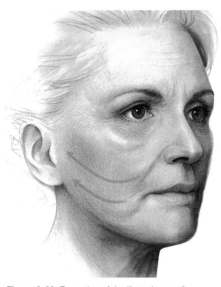

Figure 2-20: Formation of the "lateral sweep"

Youthful Eyes Stay Youthful

The Composite Facelift restores the original luster of your eye region with a new twist on the standard blepharoplasty. In 1995 I published the original article on preserving the fat of the lower eyelid instead of the old practice of removing it. Three years later I added the "septal reset" to the procedure, to not only preserve the under-eye fat, but to reset it along with its firm cover (the septum) to a position over the orbital bone. This

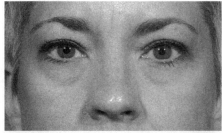

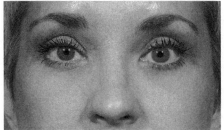

Figure 2-21: Before and after a Composite Facelift. The septal reset creates a smooth transition between lower eyelid and cheek.

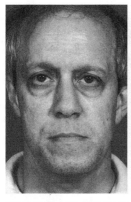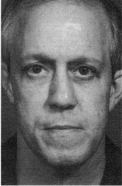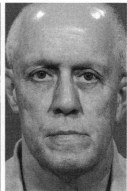

Figure 2-22: Long-term results: Left, before septal reset. Center, one year later. Right, 15 years after surgery.

creates a natural transition between the soft under-eye tissue and your cheekbone **(Figure 2-21)**.

The septal reset was the "even better" operation I advanced in 1996 and republished in 2004. I am now seeing patients with excellent results that are still stable after twelve years **(Figures 2-22 and 2-23)**. This maneuver not only remedies the gaunt or hollow appearance of the eye socket

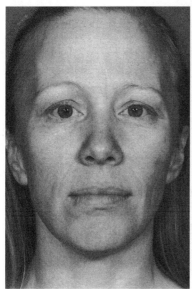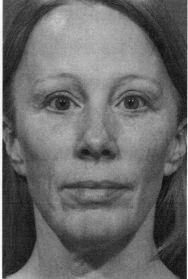

Figure 2-23: This younger patient did not need a complete facelift for rejuvenation. Left: Before surgery. Right: Ten years after a browlift, upper blepharoplasty, and septal reset.

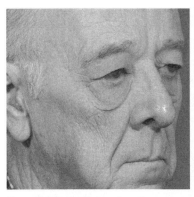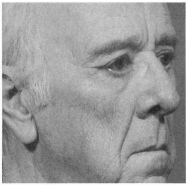

Figure 2-24: Left: "Festoons" are the most severe form of orbicularis muscle excess. Right: Orbicularis repositioning with the septal reset delivers a handsome change, even without a complete facelift.

that we often see with traditional facelifts, but also removes the signs of aging apparent anytime we can see the bony anatomy underneath the eyes. Moreover, since part of the procedure involves lifting and repositioning the orbicularis muscle, the septal reset prevents your face from being marred by the muscle bulge of the malar crescent. (Refer to Figure 2-12). It can even remedy festoons, the most severe form of orbicularis muscle excess **(Figure 2-24)**.

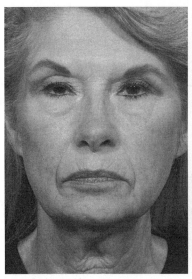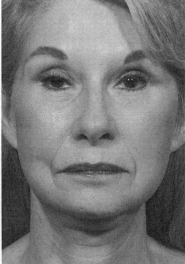

Figure 2-25: Before Composite and one year after. The septal reset smoothes the eye-cheek junction. (Any degree of facial asymmetry will be the same following surgery.)

Correcting this area not only restores your eye's smooth contour, but also gives you an attractive upper cheek **(Figure 2-25)**, with the "seamless" transition between eyelid and cheek found in youth. Most important for this youthful appearance is the high position of the "cheek mass" that is the highlight of your cheek, and the biggest contributor to your facial harmony and beauty. This is a consistent and unique feature of the Composite Facelift.

The Forehead: An Extra Measure of Lift

As the tissues of the cheek are lifted, they impact the tissues of the temple, which must then be moved in the same direction (vertically) as the cheek. A forehead lift is, therefore, an essential part of the Composite to prevent a bunching of skin to the side of the eyes. By repositioning and tightening the forehead, other signs of aging in the upper face — droopy eyebrows, "hooded" eyelids, and forehead furrows — are eliminated **(Figures 2-26, 2-27)**.

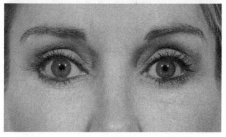

Figure 2-26: The corrugator muscles cause those frown lines. Removing them is part of the Composite procedure.

Do you look like you're constantly frowning? Those vertical lines above your nose are caused by two small muscles called the corrugators. Surgically removing them eliminates that worried look. These muscles are also the most popular target for BOTOX® injections. BOTOX® works well, but must be repeated every three to four months. Removing the muscles ensures those frown lines are gone forever.

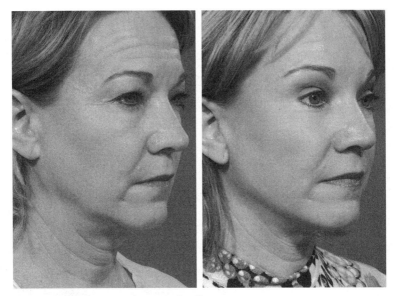

Figure 2-27: Before and after Composite Facelift.

Incorporating a brow lift with the Composite does more than just do away with the worried, concerned look. By raising the forehead vertically, your surgeon anchors the upper most part of your face so it won't descend faster than your other features. When performed with other Composite maneuvers, the brow lift helps eliminate facial distortions while ensuring a pleasing, overall even look. Disharmony may result if the forehead lift is not done, and a youthful facelift is observed under an aging forehead.

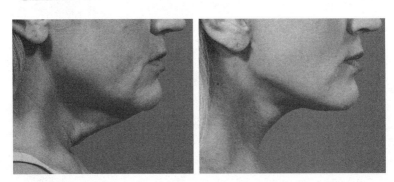

Figure 2-28: Loose skin and muscle are tightened.

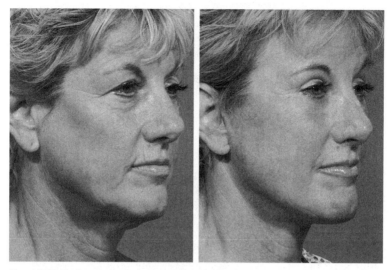

Figure 2-29: Necks vary greatly, but can always be improved.

Sticking Your Neck Out

The neck lift is part of every Composite Facelift and is never omitted. Individual neck anatomy varies greatly, but it can always be improved **(Figures 2-28, 29, 30)**. If the neck fat is too thick, it is reduced to a

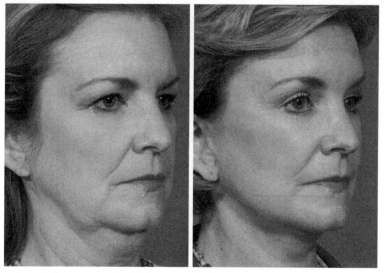

Figure 2-30: Excess fat is reduced to a normal level.

normal level. Some patients have no extra fat, but have prominent bands of platysma muscle visible at the front of the neck. I always tell patients that the neck changes are never as impressive as the face since the skin of the neck is positioned over a "hinge joint" and, like the knee and elbow, this elastic skin may look tight or loose depending on the way you tilt your head in flexion or extension.

The *Do-Over*: Revising Previous Facelifts

The beauty of the Composite Facelift is that we can apply the same principles to correcting facial distortions as we do to prevent them in the first place. For more than a decade, I've been able to demonstrate to most patients that windswept pulls and other facial distortions from previous surgery can be markedly improved **(Figure 2-31)**.

I am often reminded of the old saying, "If Plan A doesn't work the first time, don't make Plan B the same as Plan A." In facial rejuvenation, traditional procedures are often both Plan A and B. Unfortunately, repeating a SMAS procedure can reinforce the sweep and other distortions of the first surgery. This is why patients with a history of several facelifts often look more pulled than they did after their first procedure. Many aging actors illustrate this premise; the proof is etched in every re-emphasized pull of their faces on camera.

The Composite Facelift, however, gives patients and their surgeons an option that works so well the first time in preventing facial stigmata that they aren't likely to have to return for many years. When this unique operation is used to correct the issues of past operations, it's a very successful Plan B.

During this surgery, we manipulate the skin and underlying tissues to improve an earlier outcome in the same way we initially rejuvenate the face. The Composite reverses the progressive downward movement of the cheek fat and muscle by returning them to their original position. In doing

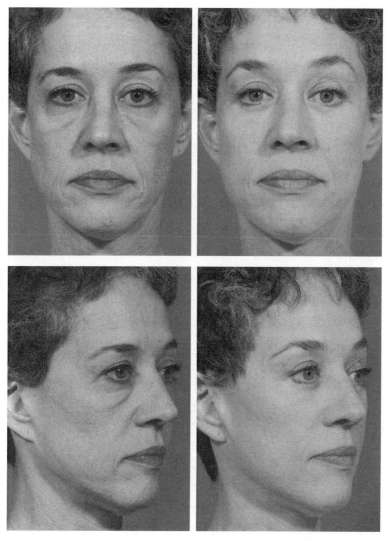

Figure 2-31: The "before" photos (left) show the results of an aging conventional facelift. The photos on the right show the improvement achieved with the Composite. *More in Chapter 4.*

so, the procedure not only corrects the imbalance of the face but also eliminates the windswept nature of those lower cheeks.

Secondly, the Composite corrects the gaunt or hollow eye created during a previous surgery by repositioning the remaining orbital fat so the eye socket has the necessary padding.

Thirdly, the Composite corrects the bulges of the croissant-shaped ridge we call the malar crescent by lifting and moving the lower eyelid muscle up toward the eye, bringing with it the malar fat that creates the higher cheek mass.

I have been able to help the majority of patients who have come to me unhappy about the long-term results of previous facial surgery. Whether they have been through one operation or many, I am happy say that they enjoy a beautiful, longer lasting result after revision surgery. My philosophy is that I will never agree to do revision surgery unless I can assure the patient of significant improvement. Surgery is never 100% perfect, and the need for small touch-ups is always possible. Patients understand this, and the limitations of surgery, if they have been sufficiently educated and have asked all the right questions. *(Read more about the Composite as revision surgery in Part Three.)*

The Whole Package: Combining Procedures

Other procedures—additional face procedures and body work—can be combined with a Composite Facelift. The Composite Facelift is typically performed in an accredited hospital or surgery center under general anesthesia, so we can add other procedures safely and effectively. You must discuss this with your surgeon, however, since not every patient is a good candidate for combined procedures and not every surgeon is comfortable doing it.

I often incorporate a chin implant, for instance, to help balance the lower face. This can significantly improve the profile by giving dimension to a receding chin. Cheek implants, however, are an entirely different story. Since the Composite repositions the fat of the mid-face area to its youthful standing, we never have to rely on cheek implants. In fact, I find their presence to be too "angular" and unnatural and almost always remove them when performing a Composite Facelift on a patient who has them from previous surgery.

Rhinoplasty (reshaping the nose) is often requested, and can deliver predictably good results. Many of my facelift patients complete their new look with breast surgery or other body work at the same time or a later date. *(See Part 4 – Complementary Procedures)*

Are You A Good Candidate For The Composite?

If you are a good candidate for facial rejuvenation, you are likely a good candidate for this procedure **(Figures 2-32 through 2-35)**.

A Composite Facelift may be right for you if aging is noticeable in all parts of your face. In short, just about everyone from their late 40s on is a good candidate, as most of us age evenly after that point. This means that just a little nip-and-tuck will not give the desired result. The best plan is a completely freshened look from hairline to neck.

A conventional facelift can still yield beautiful, satisfying results if you're younger or if you have what cosmetic surgeons call a "positive vector orbit." That is, if you have inherited the youthfully smooth lower-eye-to-

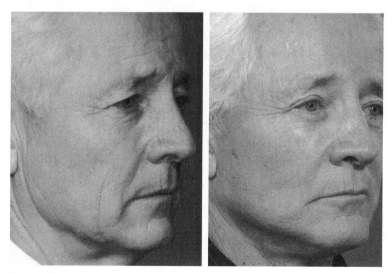

Figure 2-32: Excess fat is reduced to a normal level.

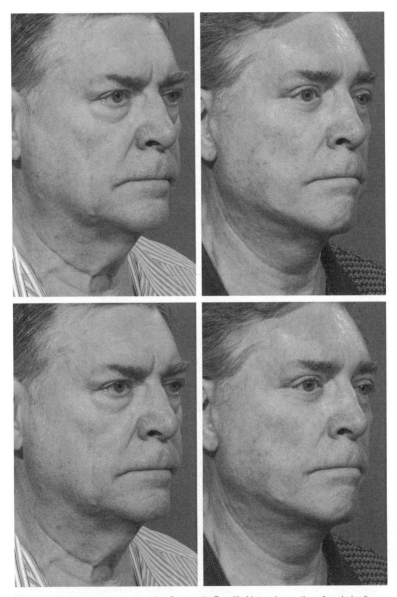

Figure 2-33: Before and one year after Composite Facelift. Note rejuvenation of neck, jawline, cheek, eye and forehead. All endpoints were achieved.

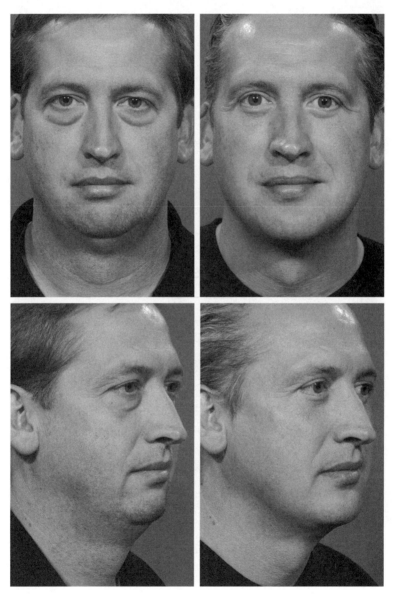

Figure 2-34: Before and one year after surgery. For this younger patient, an upper blepharoplasty, cheek lift (which included the septal reset), chin implant, and reduction of neck fat gave the desired result.

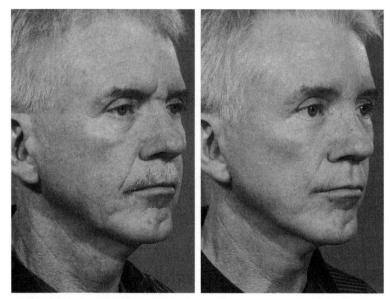

Figure 2-35: Before and one year after a Composite Facelift.

cheek contours that make Clint Eastwood look younger than springtime, a standard approach may make your day. If, on the other hand, you have Al Pacino's obvious malar crescent (excess orbicularis muscle) in your genes, you are better suited for a Composite Facelift. It will dispense with your sags and bulges, and regardless of whether you are male or female, you can achieve excellent results. I have performed thousands of Composite Facelifts on both men and women to their great satisfaction and mine. Whatever your gender, you must meet the same health criteria demanded of any such surgical procedure. *(See Part 4 – Medical History and Physical Exam)*

FAQs About The Composite Lift

How long does a Composite Lift take?

The Composite Facelift usually takes about four hours to perform and is done with a light general anesthesia. The length of time a surgeon takes to do the surgery varies with each individual surgeon and does not impact the end result. Only your safety and the final outcome are the important factors.

Where should it be performed?

I feel strongly that this surgery should be performed in an accredited hospital or surgery center under general anesthesia, with an overnight stay.

How long is the recovery?

You will likely undergo a longer convalescence than with a conventional facelift. This technique carries the same general risks, such as blood clots and nerve damage, as standard procedures. Since the Composite requires extensive work around the eyes, you may experience additional bruising and swelling in that area. I always tell my patients that if they have an in-your-face job, they probably will have to wait about six weeks to take on the world with a socially acceptable look. I advise mothers of the bride to allow eight to ten weeks. Otherwise, most people can be out and about within three to four weeks. Tinted glasses cover eyelid swelling, and many of my out-of-town patients feel comfortable flying home after five days.

When will I see the final result?

Improvements continue to be seen for up to a year as healing becomes complete. Traditional facelifts, on the other hand, offer a quicker return to social activities with minimal bruising and swelling. Although you can be up and about in just two to three weeks, you run the risk of long-term disappointment. With the Composite Facelift procedure, the more you have done, the longer the healing, but also the more impressive and durable the results.

How Long Will A Composite Facelift Last?

Over the decade that I have performed this procedure, I have seen a remarkable stability in every portion of the face. Whether it is a first-time facelift or a second-time effort, we have demonstrated in follow-up studies that the modifications to the forehead, mid-face and lower face regions change very little. Moreover, because the areas retain their relationship to each other, the characteristic distortions of other lifts simply do not develop. The face continues the normal dynamic descent of aging in a pleasing, balanced way. We have, after all, only turned back the clock, not completely stopped it!

Is the Composite Facelift the ultimate facial rejuvenation procedure? Hardly, but I think of it as one step in many that aesthetic surgeons are taking to achieve outstanding results. No doubt there will be better techniques evolving as time goes on. When I first published it, the Composite Facelift represented the first major change in rejuvenation surgery in many years. Additional approaches have come along as many surgeons strive to achieve similar results. Many work very well. On the other hand, if the emphasis on quick and inexpensive procedures continues, there will be fewer surgeons interested in learning to do advanced facelifts. Presently there seems to be a step backward towards the modified short scar facelifts that were popular many years ago. It will be a shame if fewer surgeons are trained to correct facial surgery problems while there are more problems being created.

With the Composite, I have been able to correct scores of faces marked by previous procedures or just the passage of time. I recall one patient who felt that he was so deformed by multiple past surgeries that he asked for an initial appointment after office hours, so my other patients would not mistakenly think I did his original surgeries. No one should walk away from facelift surgery feeling so badly about the way they look.

Thanks to this technique, we can now restore the facial harmony of youth. ❖

FOR FIRST-TIME PATIENTS:
10 Questions to Ask Your Surgeon

1. Do you do a Composite Facelift, including the septal reset and orbicularis repositioning?

2. If you don't do the Composite Facelift, what technique will you use and why?

3. How will you create a smooth transition between my cheekbone and lower eyelid? Do you do it with injections? If so, what material do you use, and how long will it last?

4. Can you show me photographs of your patients that show how the elevated cheek fat now blends with the lower eyelid?

5. Do you do the open or endoscopic forehead lift technique? Can you lower my hairline if it is too high?

6. Are any touch-ups typically needed with the facelift procedure you do? If so, what are they? What is your policy regarding additional surgical fees?

7. If I have the Composite procedure, what are the chances that you will need to do a corrective surgery down the road? How long will the results of my facelift last?

8. If you don't do the Composite Facelift, how do you prevent the lateral sweep of my cheeks?

9. Do you do a formal cheek lift? What happens if the eyelid gets pulled down? Can you correct it?

10. How long does the surgery take? Where is it performed and under what type of anesthesia?

PART THREE

PROBLEMS WITH TODAY'S FACELIFTS

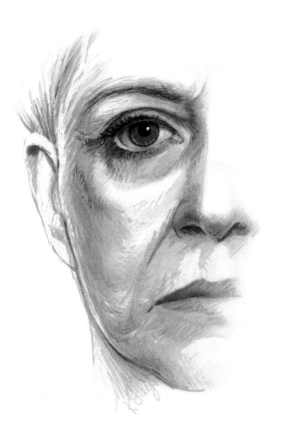

*A facelift should give people a look
that grows old gracefully*

Shouldn't your facelift age well? After all, you've invested time, effort and considerable resources to rejuvenate your features and update your look. You'd certainly like the new image in your mirror to last months, if not years. But what happens when your long-term expectations are met only by short-term results? The truth is, the same facelift procedures that yield fabulous new profiles right after surgery can fade and distort before your next birthday. You may be wondering how this can happen, given the technological advances in all of plastic surgery. The reality is that the most popular techniques, which have been done for years, are falling woefully short over time. I know. I used to do them. I see the results every day both in my office and everywhere I go. An early pleasing result frequently gives way to that "facelifted" look that everyone would rather avoid. And disappointments continue with the "minimally invasive" procedures currently being promoted, simply because so little is done.

I believe that anyone who is unhappy with a previous facelift would surely want to get it corrected if they knew that it could be easily done, and if they knew who to go to. I even see it on some of my friends, but it is impossible for me to tell them about this new operation unless they come to my office and ask for my advice. Most will either go through life looking the same, or they will get another lift just like the first, which only reinforces the "facelifted look." The potential for reclaiming their youthful beauty is never fully realized.

Why Facelift Patients Are Often Dissatisfied

Each year I meet hundreds of men and women who want me to give them back the faces of their youth. Many are visiting a cosmetic surgeon for the first time. They have thought long and hard about how lifting their wrinkling skin and sagging features might also elevate their confidence and restore their self-esteem. They are anxious to match the vision they see in the mirror with the young and vibrant person they feel they still are inside. I am excited to help them.

Many people who come to me, however, aren't so optimistic. They once had the same enthusiasm for a plastic surgeon's scalpel and skill as every facelift newcomer. But they have seen the immediate, meticulous results of their surgeon's work fade over time. Perhaps you recognize it in your own face: there's no longer the youthful harmony you enjoyed right after surgery. Instead, your lower cheeks and jawline remain tight while other areas, such as your upper cheeks and forehead, continue to fall. You see the pulls and tensions across your face, and often notice the look of a "pulled mouth." The area under your eyes takes on a hollow, even gaunt look, leaving you with a classic mask-like appearance.

The natural reaction is to blame the surgeon. But most cosmetic surgeons are extremely capable of bringing home a beautiful, youthful contour that satisfies your vision and refreshes your looks. Blame the technique, not the surgeon.

It was not the surgeon, but the traditional old-fashioned technique that led to your current appearance.

What happened? Some slippage can be explained by the normal process of aging. None of us can halt the inevitable march of time. But it's not always the passage of years that makes individuals unhappy about their outcomes. I've spent the better part of my cosmetic surgery career helping people disillusioned about their looks. What I have learned, by treating thousands of men and women, is that today's facelifts often don't perform well in the long run because of the very techniques we have come to rely on as surgeons. These are the techniques I was trained to do 35 years ago, and are still being done universally by many of the world's most famous surgeons.

Traditional Techniques: The Problem

Conventional facelifts have changed little over the past 40 years. Actually, they have changed very little in concept since the 1920s, when the earliest techniques were published. The simplest operation, still done today by some of the most well known surgeons, is the *skin lift*. This is simply a technique where the surgeon first lifts and then redrapes the skin of the face, as you would redrape a bedspread. It gives the "rested" appearance surgeons have bragged about for years. Compared to some of the impressive results achieved today with newer techniques, though, it changes the appearance only minimally. The duration is variable, but the most frequent complaint is the brief time of looking good. Many patients are disappointed because there was so little improvement and it didn't last. This might be acceptable if it only did little good but did not have the potential for creating problems as time goes by. But there is never a guarantee that you won't develop an unwanted appearance, and there is no objective way for the surgeon or you to know that ahead of time.

The SMAS Facelift

As an acronym for *superficial musculoaponeurotic system*, SMAS not only refers to the most common conventional facelift performed today but also to a significant part of your lower facial anatomy. The SMAS is the soft connective and fatty tissue layers directly below the skin, and the muscle (platysma) that it envelops.

Since the introduction of the SMAS procedure in the 1970s, standard facelifts have consisted largely of repositioning the sagging muscles under the lower cheek and neck and tightening the overlying skin. The rest of the deeper tissues of the face, however, remain untouched.

There is no question that the SMAS has been thought to be a significant improvement over the skin-only facelift. Although both approaches call for lifting tissue in the same single direction towards the ear

(Figure 3-1), the SMAS was an important step in our quest to provide men and women with the most natural appearance possible by going deeper than just the surface. It was the first time a structure under the skin was manipulated during a facelift. Without doubt, the jawline was

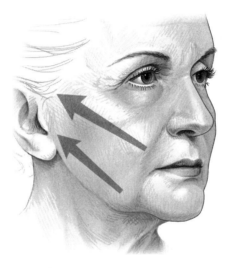

Figure 3-1: Both skin-only and SMAS procedures lift only towards the ear

smoothed out, but the underlying tissues of the *upper* face stayed undisturbed. Like all surgeons, I was enthusiastic, but after observing so many patients over the years, I came to the conclusion that the effect of the SMAS procedure is actually too enduring, and thus contributes to disharmony as the rest of the face ages.

Through the years, the SMAS has prompted many variations, including the *Deep Plane Facelift,* my own next-step attempt to improve on the traditional technique. But even with other surgeons fine-tuning the SMAS procedure, many patients were still being disillusioned with their long-term results.

Let's take a closer look at how this traditional technique works.

The SMAS facelift is based on the concept that facial sagging is more than just a superficial problem. It's actually caused by the face's underlying structures, including the SMAS layers, losing their tone and falling, pulling the skin with them. Outwardly, the cheeks become hollow, the jawline develops jowls, and the vertical creases (nasolabial folds) between the nose and corners of the mouth deepen.

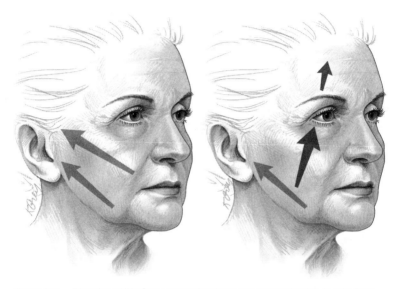

Figure 3-2 — Direction of lift: Only a lateral direction in conventional facelifts, but the Composite adds a strong vertical vector.

During a SMAS procedure, the surgeon lifts and tightens the underlying structures of the lower face and neck (the platysma muscle) before repositioning the skin in a separate maneuver. Both layers are pulled in a lateral or sideways direction toward the ears. This is classified as a *lateral vector facelift* (**Figure 3-2**). As for other parts of the face, the forehead isn't usually included and the eyes are an optional separate procedure. Doctors may or may not perform a blepharoplasty, an upper and lower eyelid lift. When given the choice, patients may skip the eyelid surgery for cost or other reasons, since a surgeon can perform a SMAS facelift without doing the lower eyelid.

By addressing deeper tissues, the SMAS seemed to alleviate the severe facial tension that resulted from just stretching the skin without repositioning what's underneath. Indeed, because it turns jowls into a tightened jawline that stays youthfully in place, this procedure remains the facial rejuvenation gold standard for most surgeons around the world.

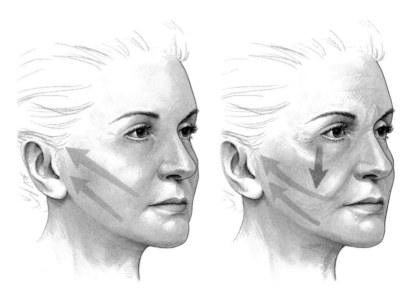

Figure 3-3 — The Aging Conventional Facelift: Lateral direction of pull in conventional facelifts. On the right: unsupported tissues of the upper face fall as aging continues.

Why Doesn't The SMAS Work Long-Term?

The SMAS facelift doesn't perform well in the long run largely because of problems inherent in the operation itself. As we have seen, it does an excellent job of creating a tighter jawline and firmer neck. It even addresses the tension on the skin by repositioning the structures underneath. But by not lifting the upper cheeks and forehead vertically, these parts of the face are free to continue their natural descent. By only pulling the tissues of the lower face sideways, everything but the jawline is left ripe for future sagging **(Figure 3-3)**. Even when the under-eye area is addressed, the eye socket can eventually sink, leaving a concave or hollow contour sitting atop sagging cheek fat and eyelid muscles, which sit atop a taut jawline.

Together, these events often lead to the characteristic pulls, tension, and "facelifted" appearance we can see in far too many people. It doesn't happen with every patient — depending on age, skin and anatomy, many individuals experience very acceptable long-term results with traditional procedures. If you are in your early to mid-40s, with little drooping, for instance, you can enjoy beautiful outcomes for years before there may be any inkling (if at all) that you might need additional work. Even if your face shows significant sagging, chances are you will be excited about your initial result. But as gravity takes hold, and your picture-perfect face starts descending, you are likely to see a mature profile that lacks the harmony of your youth. The unevenness manifests itself in the mirror.

Because SMAS techniques have become almost an obligatory part of the international culture of facelift surgery, I am sure that they will continue to be performed by the vast majority of surgeons. Almost all of the surgeons responsible for organizing scientific meetings and teaching aesthetic surgery to plastic surgeons are SMAS enthusiasts. It would be impossible for them to suddenly change a philosophy so ingrained after thirty or more years. We become "known by" what we preach at symposia. A prominent surgeon must have his original personal operation. Presentations are carefully put together after years of practice. It is not uncommon for a surgeon to give the same presentation with the same patient photos over decades if he is still advocating the same technique. Some have changed a minor portion of an existing operation and then given their new operation a marketable new title.

The same widespread acceptance of SMAS facelifts by plastic surgeons will never be replaced by a mass rejection of its value. As long as lateral vector facelifts are done, the SMAS maneuver will be popular. For those surgeons who have converted to vertical type facelifts, it has become easy to abandon the SMAS in order to achieve better results, but these surgeons are a small minority with voices rarely heard.

Let's take a look at the predictable markers that a traditional facelift procedure can leave on your face.

Facial Distortions Tell the Story

As mentioned in earlier chapters, there are three distinctive signs that your facelift is not aging well: the *lateral sweep, hollow eye,* and *malar crescent.* It may be months, perhaps even years, before you see any of these, but when they occur, they distort the image you've spent thousands to restore.

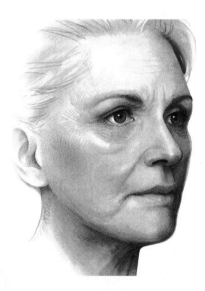

Figure 3-4 — The Lateral Sweep: The stretched look that can occur as a conventional facelift ages

Problem – The Lateral Sweep

The most obvious problem associated with a standard facelift is an expression that I coined for an article I wrote in 1998, and what surgeons now commonly refer to as a *lateral sweep*. It's the distinctive swept-back or stretched appearance between the corners of the mouth and the earlobes that tell friends and family you've definitely had some work

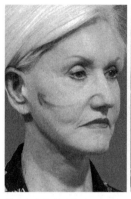 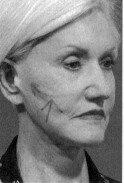 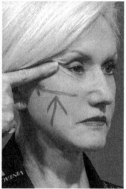

Figure 3-5: You can correct your own lateral sweep, or as a primary patient, you can give yourself great looking young cheeks and lower eyelids by pushing the cheek upward in the direction of the arrow toward the eye. This is what a Composite Facelift does. Conventional facelifts, such as the SMAS, only move tissue toward the ear.

done. Often one sees actual lines or redirected wrinkles from the mouth to the earlobe, curving down and then up, ending at the facelift incision in front of the ear. The look will be especially pronounced if you have dry, sun-damaged skin. **(Figure 3-4)**

This tautness occurs because the surgeon only lifted the lower cheeks and jawline laterally (toward the ear) and did not lift the upper cheeks and lower eyelids vertically (toward the eye). The forehead is often left untouched as well. The initial results can be stunning, but as time goes by, the upper face continues falling, in contrast to the lower face,

THE LATERAL SWEEP TEST:

❖ Draw a line [a makeup pencil will work] from your mouth or nose to the top of your ear, following the sweep.

❖ Then draw a vertical arrow from your jaw upward toward your eye.

❖ When you push in the direction of the vertical arrow, the cheek tissue is moved back on top of the cheekbone where it needs to be, as the curved line becomes straight.

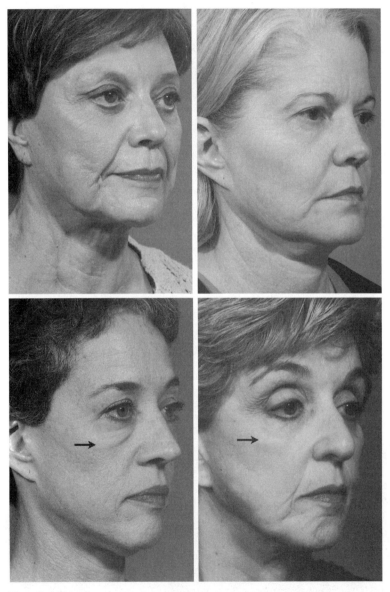

Figure 3-6: These four women all show similar signs of an aging conventional facelift. As the unsupported soft tissues of the upper face continue to age, the lateral sweep of the cheeks appears. Also note the hollow eye, and particularly in the lower photos, the malar crescent *(arrow)*.

BEFORE
AND
AFTER

PRIMARY PROCEDURES

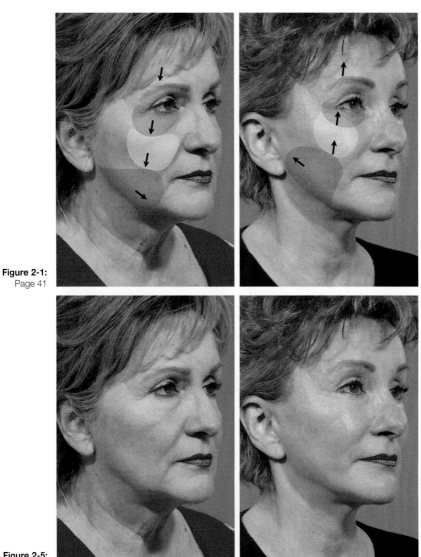

Figure 2-1:
Page 41

Figure 2-5:
Page 47

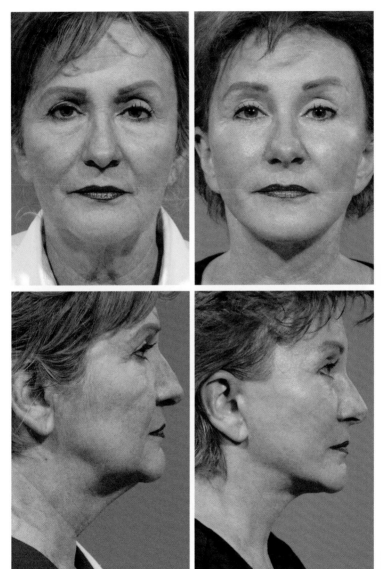

Figure 2-5:
Page 47

Figure 2-5a:
Page 48

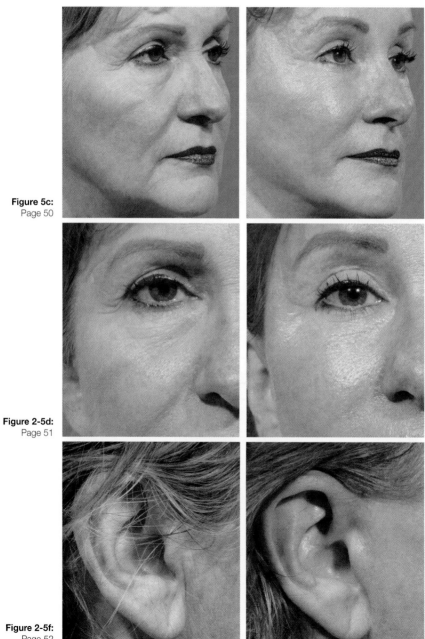

Figure 5c:
Page 50

Figure 2-5d:
Page 51

Figure 2-5f:
Page 52

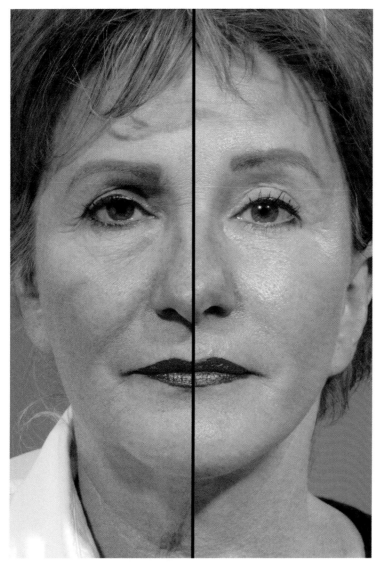

Figure 2-5g:
Page 53

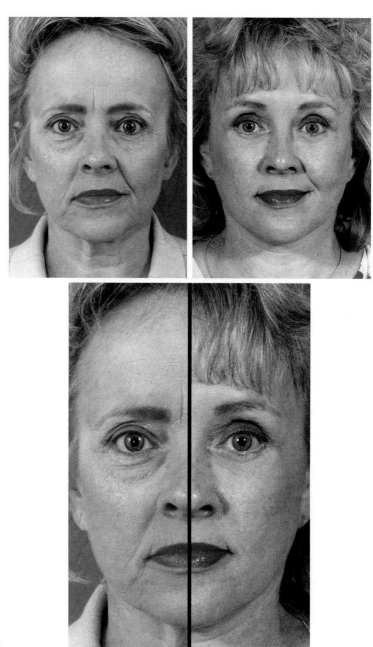

Figure 2-6:
Page 55

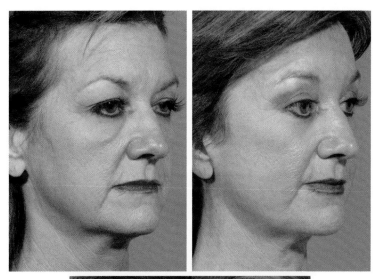

Figure 2-7:
Page 56

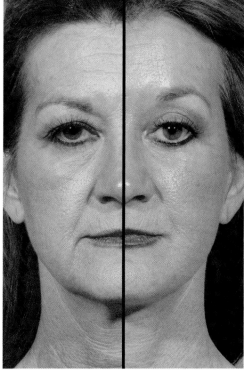

Figure 2-18:
Page 68

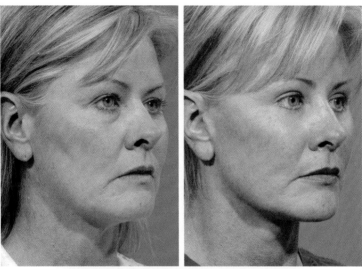

**Figures
2-8, 2-19:**
Pages 57, 69

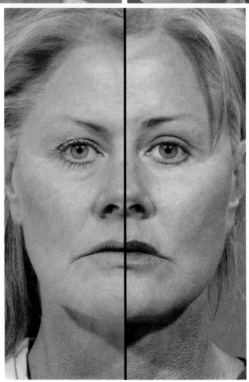

Figure 2-8:
Page 57

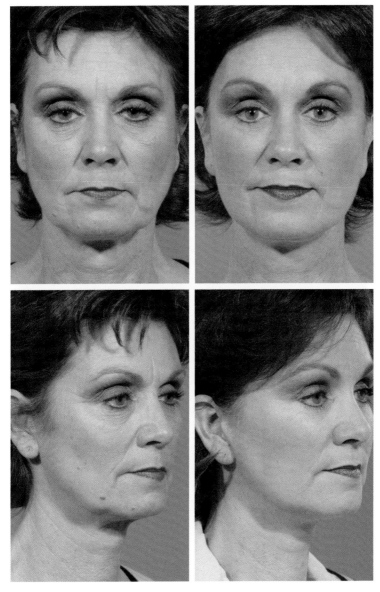

Figure 2-9:
Page 58

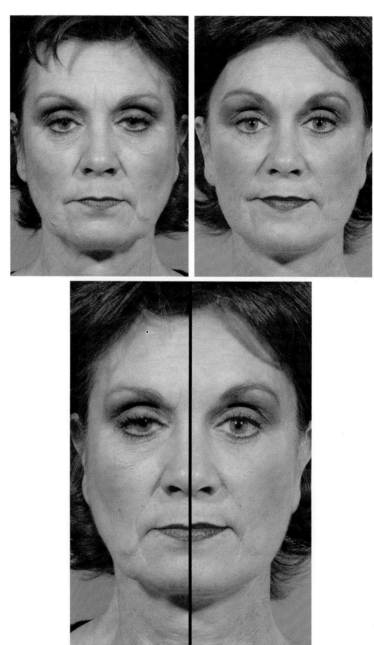

Figure 2-9

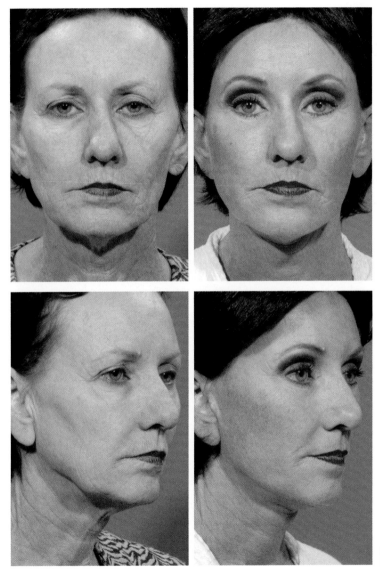

Figure 2-10:
Page 59

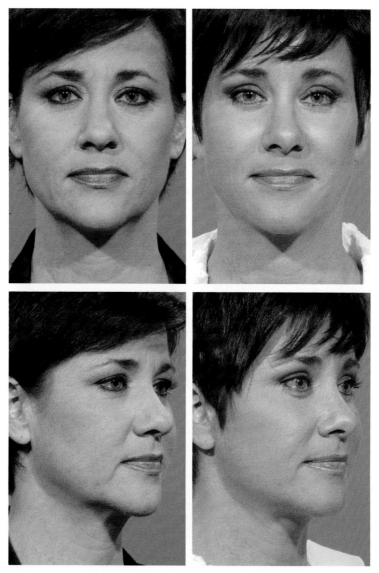

Figure 2-11:
Page 60

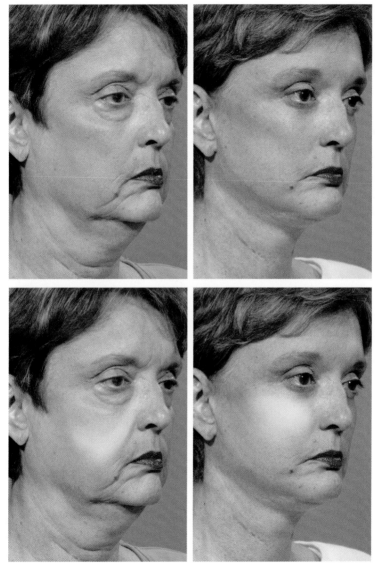

Figure 2-13:
Page 62

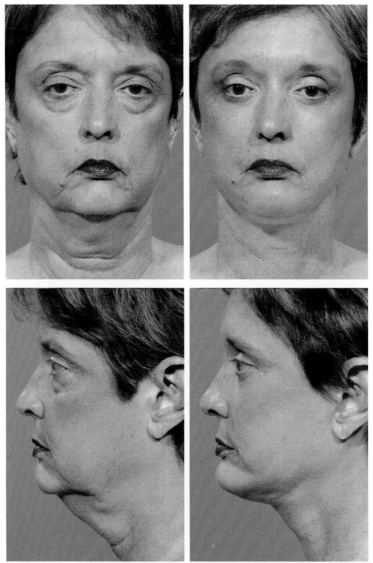

Figure 2-13

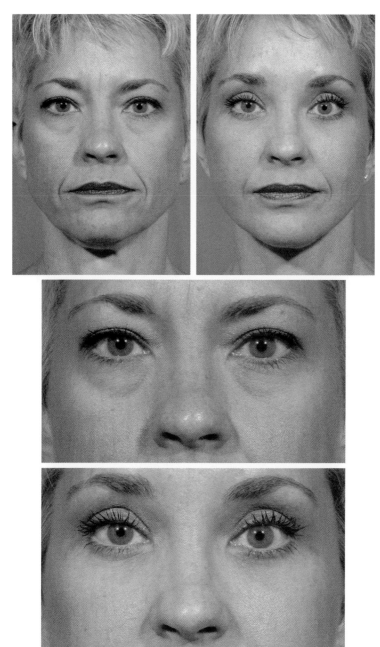

Figure 2-21:
Page 70

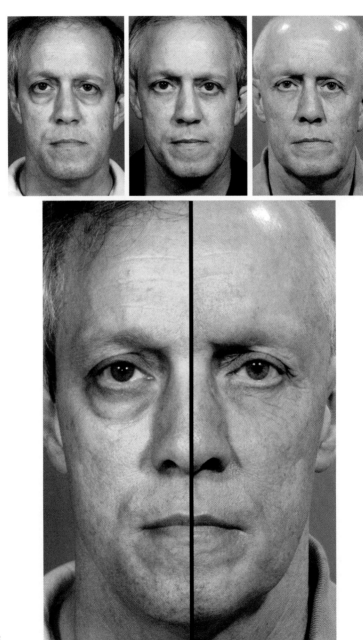

Figure 2-22:
Page 71

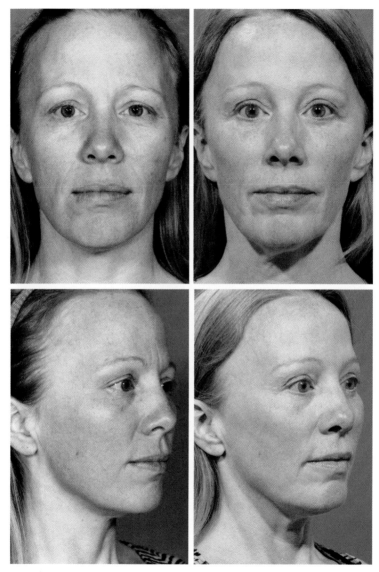

Figure 2-23:
Page 71

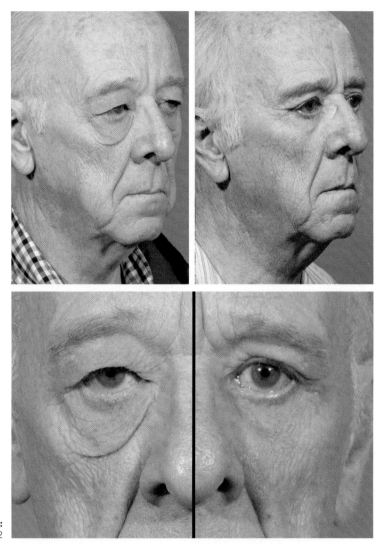

Figure 2-24:
Page 72

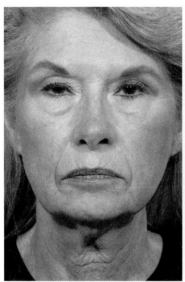
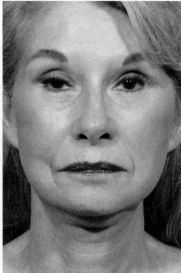

Figure 2-25:
Page 72

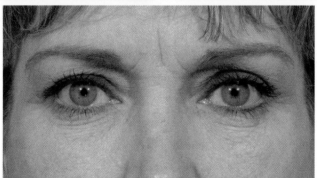

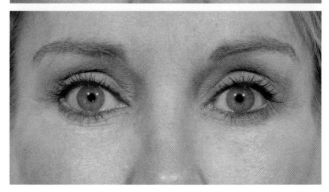

Figure 2-26:
Page 73

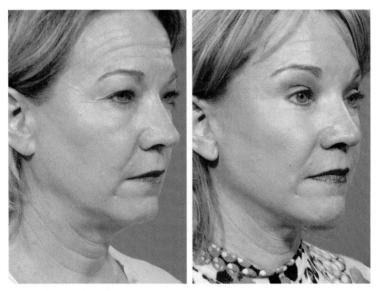

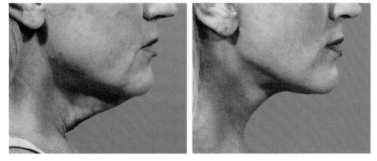

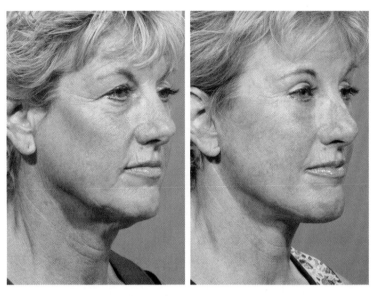

Figure 2-29:
Page 75

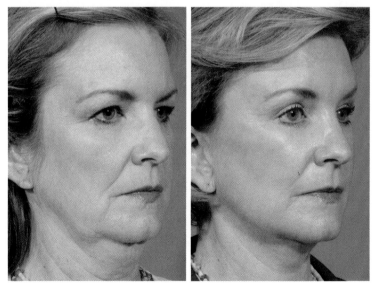

Figure 2-30:
Page 75

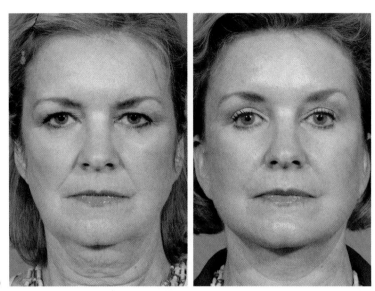

Figure 2-30

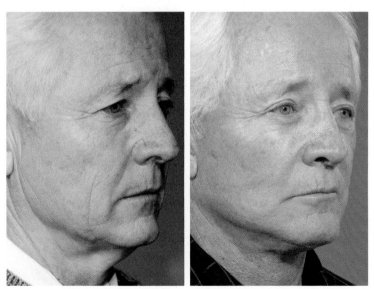

Figure 2-32:
Page 79

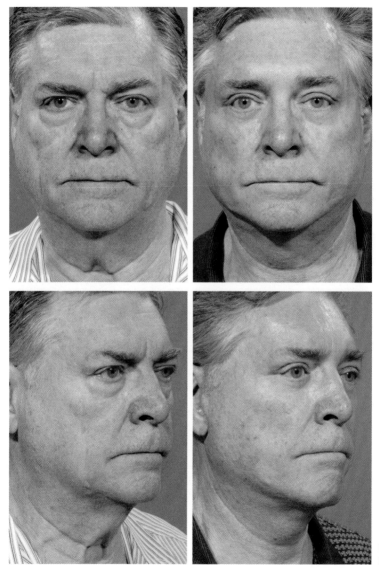

Figure 2-33:
Page 80

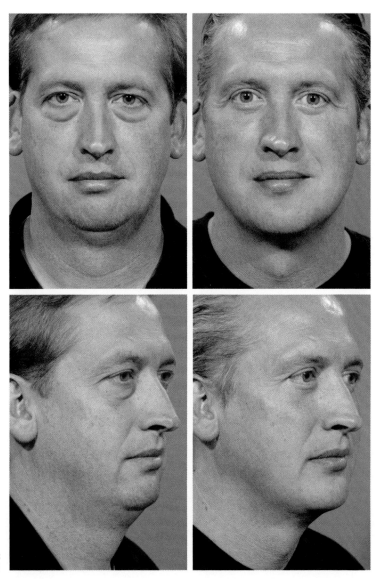

Figure 2-34:
Page 81

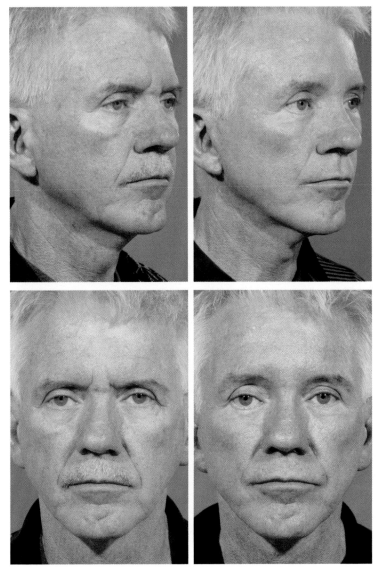

Figure 2-35:
Page 82

REVISION (SECONDARY) PROCEDURES

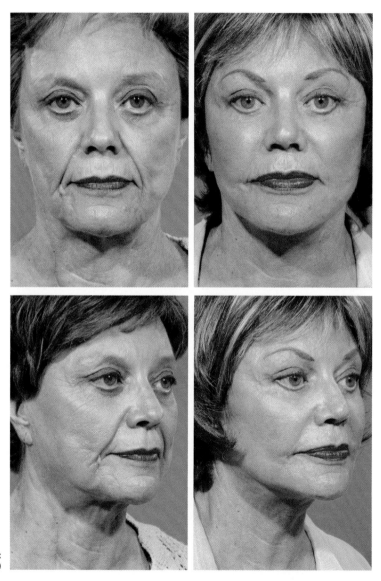

Figure 3-8:
Page 99

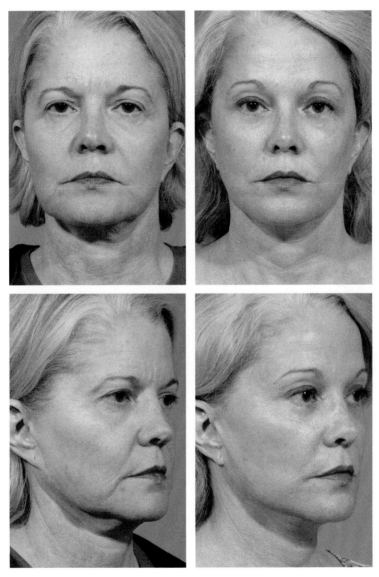

Figure 3-9:
Page 100

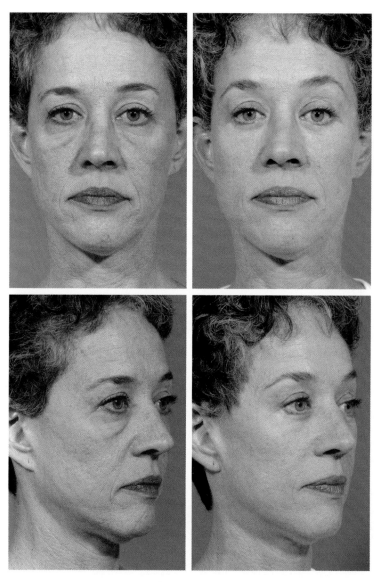

Figure 3-10:
Page 101

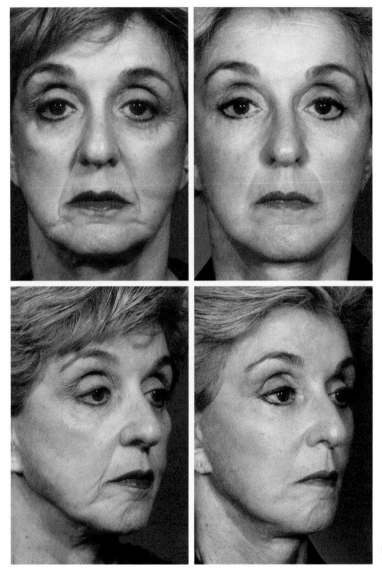

Figure 3-11:
Page 102

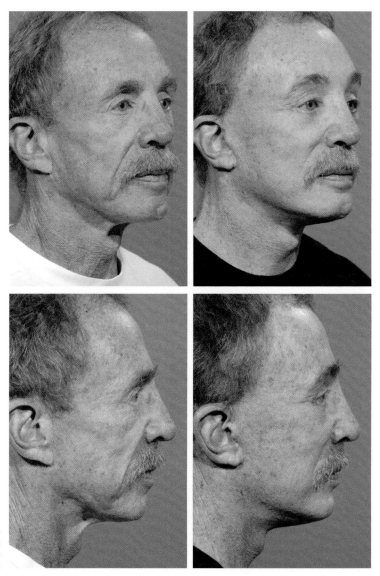

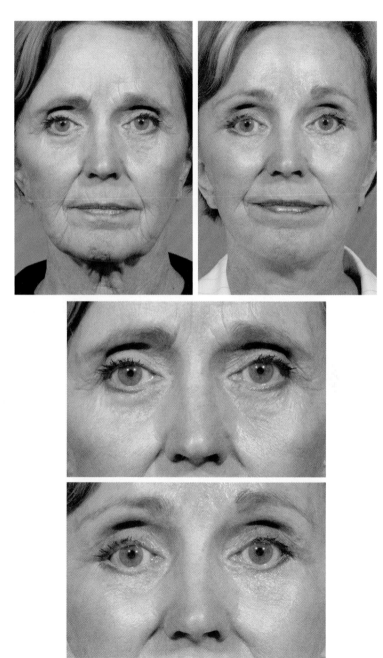

Figure 3-14:
Page 105

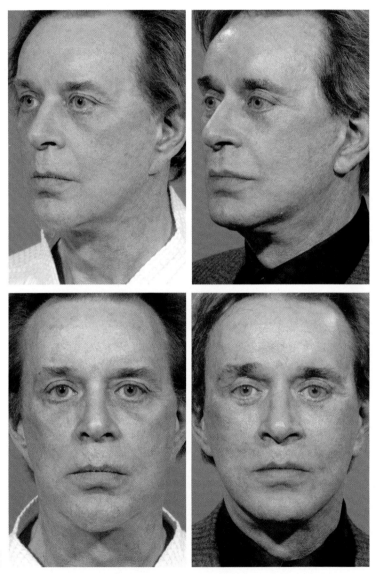

Figure 3-15:
Page 105

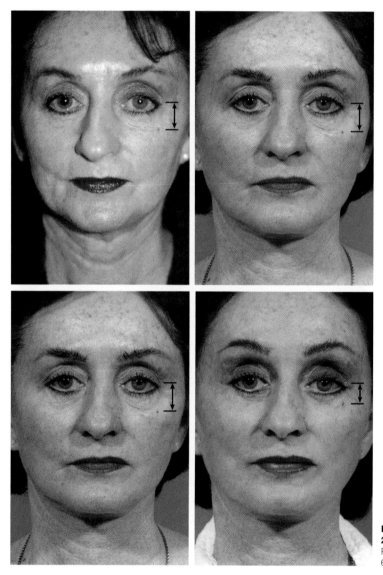

**Figures
2-15, 3-17:**
Pages
64, 65,107

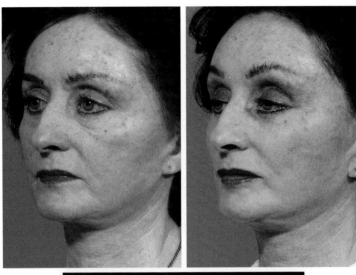

Figure 3-16:
Page 107

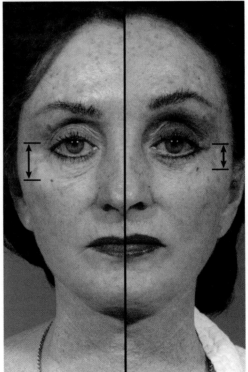

Figure 2-15c:
Page 65

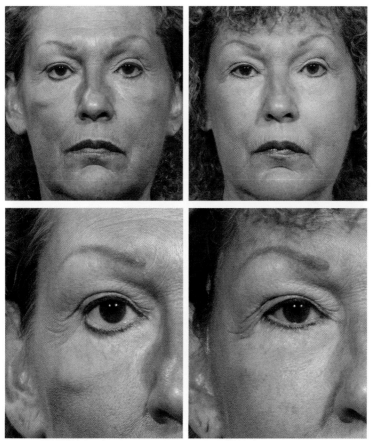

Figure 3-18:
Page 108

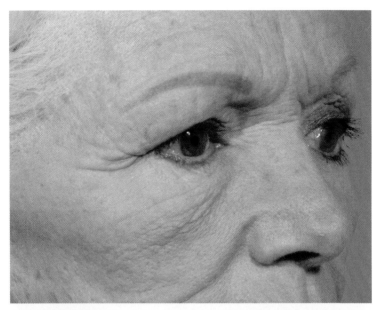

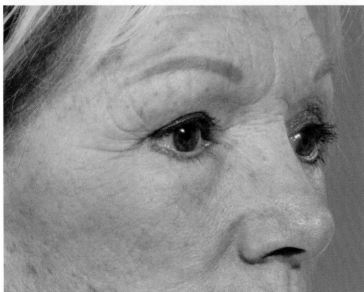

Figure 3-19:
Page 109

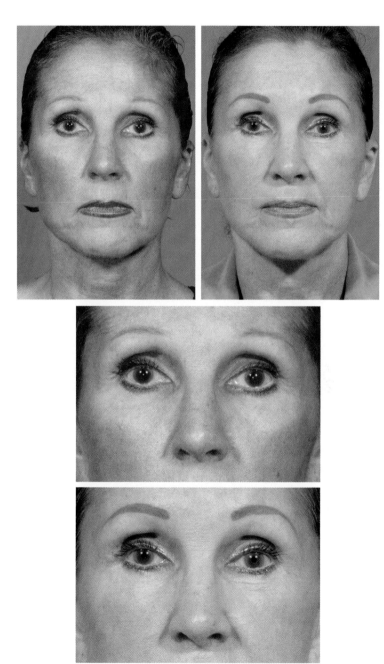

Figure 3-20
Page 109

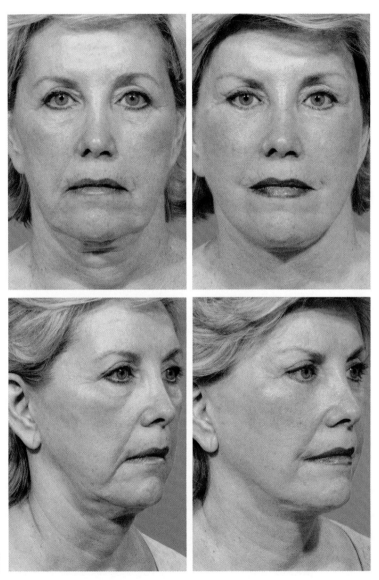

Figure 3-21:
Page 111

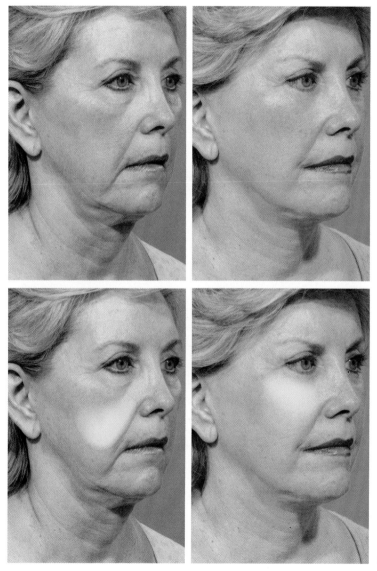

Figure 3-21

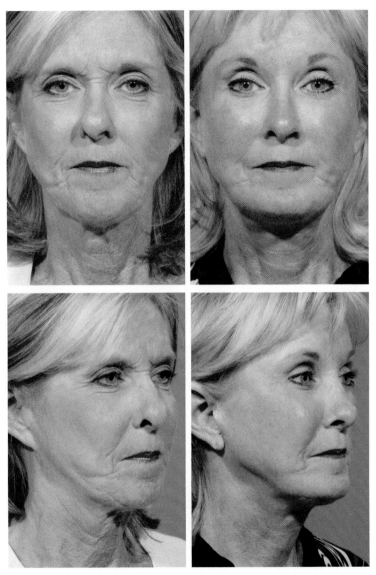

Figure 3-22:
Page 112

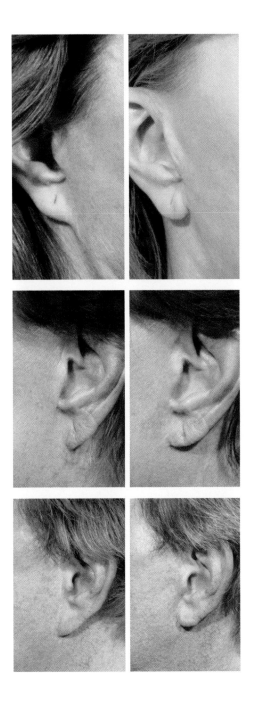

Figure 3-23:
Page 113

Figure 3-24:
Page 114

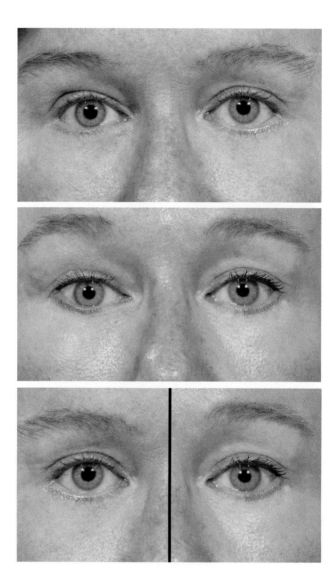

Figure 3-25:
Page 114

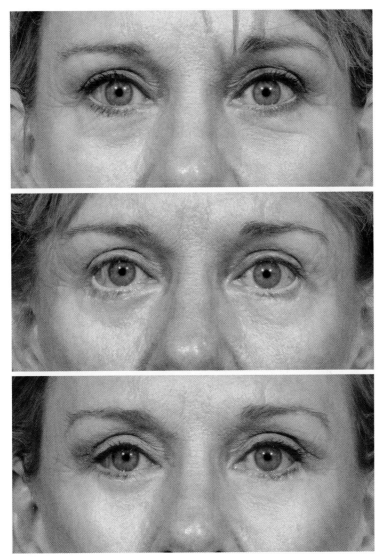

Figure 3-26:
Page 115

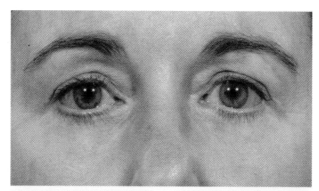

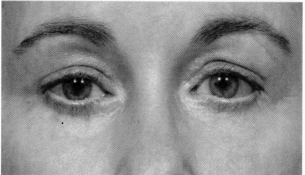

Figure 3-27:
Page 116

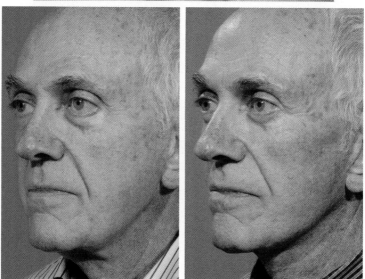

Figure 3-28:
Page 116

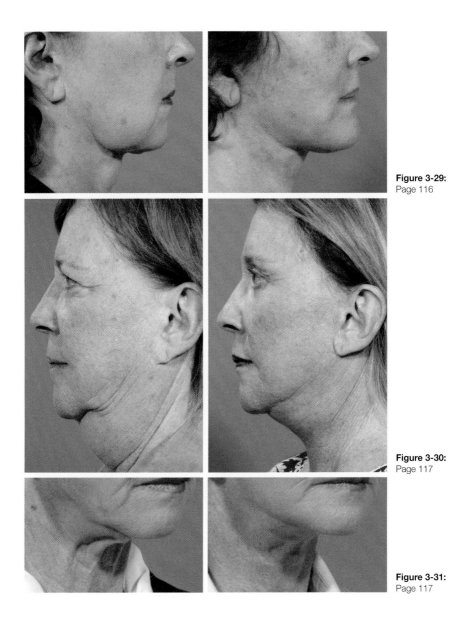

Figure 3-29:
Page 116

Figure 3-30:
Page 117

Figure 3-31:
Page 117

The Facelift Letdown

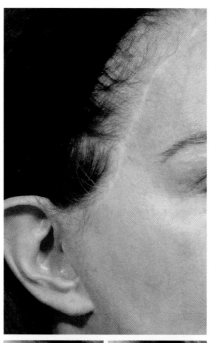

Figure 3-33:
Page 119

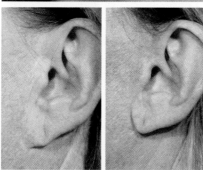

Figure 3-34:
Page 119

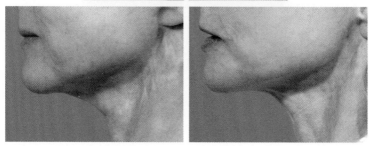

Figure 3-35:
Page 120

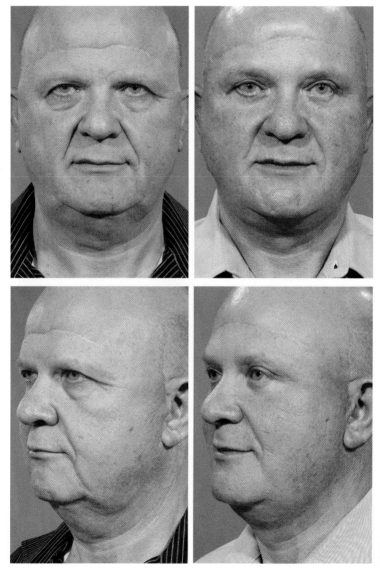

Figure 3-36:
Page 121

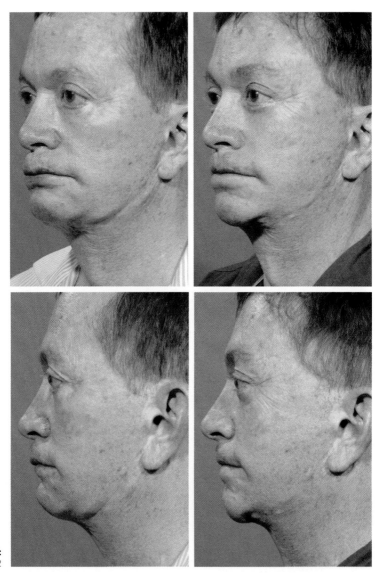

Figure 3-27:
Page 122

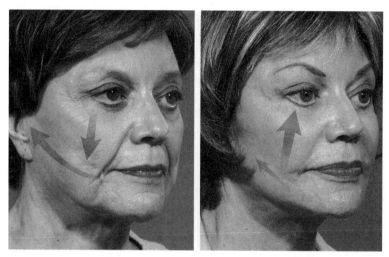

Figure 3-7: The lateral sweep is corrected by reversing the direction of movement of the cheek.

which stays taut. The fat of the cheek ("malar fat") is not supported in a vertical direction and soon starts heading south as well.

Anyone with a lateral sweep can demonstrate for themselves how it is corrected. The Composite's vertical direction of lift can be simulated by pushing your cheek up towards the eye, as seen in these photos **(Figure 3-5)**.

I noticed this in many of my own patients from the late 1980s, when I was doing the Deep Plane Facelift, repositioning both the SMAS and the cheek fat towards the ear. I published an article in 2002 on the "short-term success and long-term failure of malar fat procedures." I warned my fellow surgeons that pulling the facial tissues only in one direction is inadequate, and in fact can eventually lead to a facelift distortion. The muscle that surrounds the eye, the orbicularis, also stays undisturbed and continues showing its outline under the skin, often revealed by a crescent shape on the upper cheek. These two pieces of anatomy eventually can come crashing down on top of the taut jawline. This conflict creates a pulled mouth, tense jawline and distorted cheeks **(Figure 3-6)**.

The lateral sweep can not only get progressively worse over time, but if your surgeon uses the same traditional technique to correct it, you'll just have more of the same. It can only be corrected by reversing the direction of movement of the cheek **(Figure 3-7)**.

The following photos **(Figures 3-8 through 3-12)** show correction of the lateral sweep with a Composite Facelift.

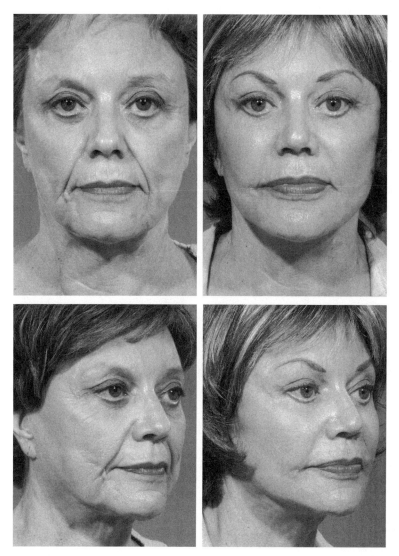

Figure 3-8: Left: After two previous conventional facelifts. Right: one year after Composite.

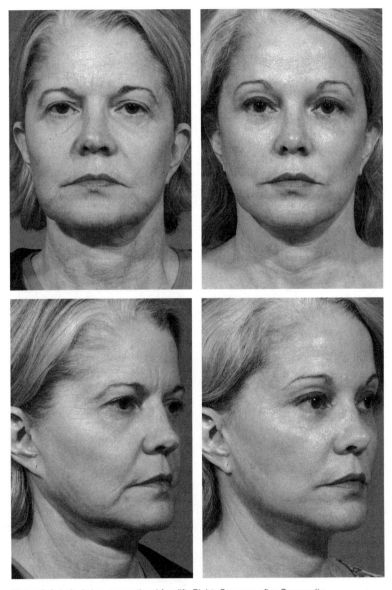

Figure 3-9: Left: Aging conventional facelift. Right: One year after Composite.

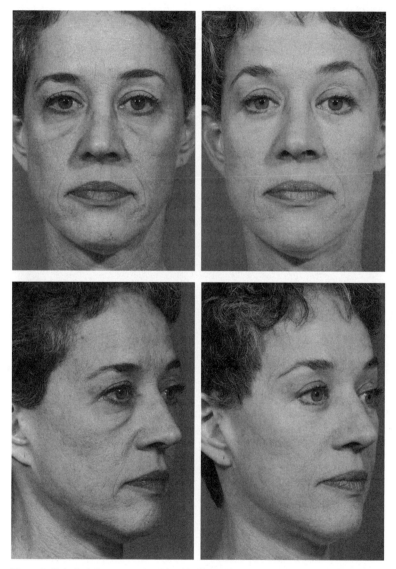

Figure 3-10: Left: Aging conventional facelift. Right: After correction with the Composite Facelift.

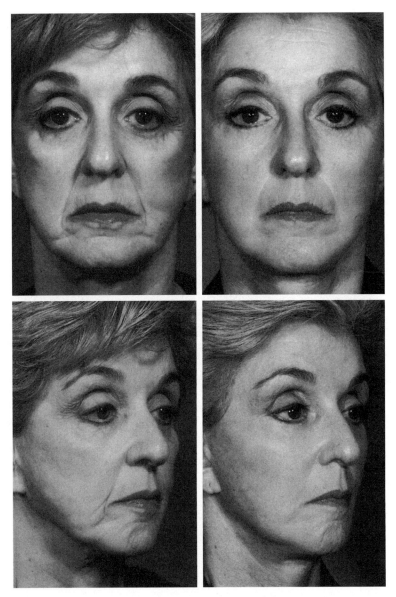

Figure 3-11: Left: Aging conventional facelift. Right: One year after Composite.

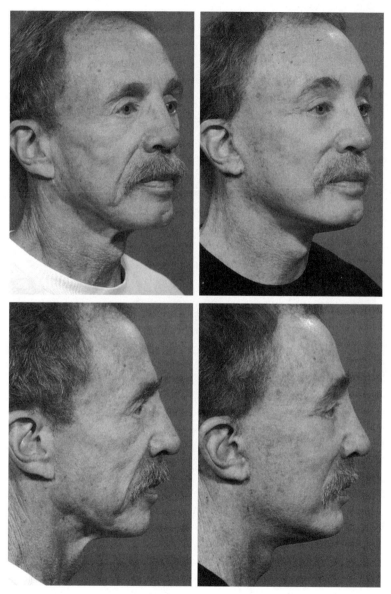

Figure 3-12: Equal opportunity: The lateral sweep happens to men as well. Left: After conventional procedure. Right: After Composite revision.

Problem – The Hollow Eye

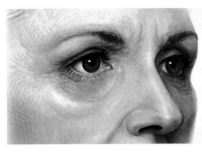

The hollow eye is a sunken or concave appearance of the eye socket. It's often associated with a traditional procedure because the surgeon has removed under-eye fat pads (the standard blepharoplasty) to eliminate the characteristic puffiness of an aging face. As we grow older, our eyelids undergo predictable changes. The skin becomes thinner, leaving the skeletal structure more pronounced and leading to a wider and deeper under-eye space. This usually begins in your 40s; the bony anatomy not seen in youth now shows up. **Figure 3-13** demonstrates this point.

In a standard facelift, surgeons typically perform a separate upper and lower eyelid lift or bypass the eye entirely. Even though restoring this area is key to achieving a soft, harmonious look, removing the fat alone often creates an even more abrupt transition between the soft lower eyelid tissue and cheekbone. The practice of removing the lower eyelid fat

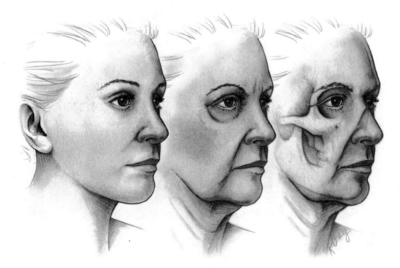

Figure 3-13: Aging leads to a "hollow" appearance of the eye.

began in 1928 in France, and is still commonly done today. I did it myself for years. But without the necessary padding, the skin may eventually collapse into a concave appearance **(Figures 3-14 and 3-15)**.

In the "septal reset" portion of the Composite Facelift, I correct this gaunt appearance by going beneath the lower eyelid, retrieving more fat and its cover (the septum), and spreading it over the hollow space onto to the cheekbone. I have never seen a hollow lower eyelid that could not be corrected, even when the earlier procedure removed a lot of fat. An added bonus is that repositioning the eyelid muscle during the cheek lift gives a thicker cover to this area. This is a good example of how all of the elements of the Composite Lift work together to rejuvenate the face. I perform a septal reset routinely in all first-time facelifts.

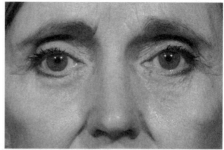
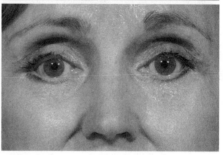

Figure 3-14: Top: After fat removal during a conventional blepharoplasty. Bottom: After Composite correction.

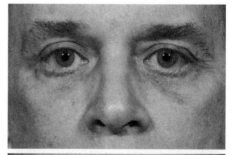
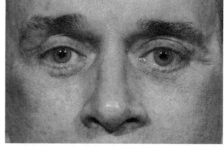

Figure 3-15: Top: Conventional blepharoplasty led to a hollow eye and scleral show. Bottom: After Composite correction.

Problem – The Malar Crescent

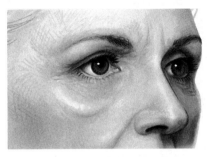

A little known part of your facial anatomy, the malar crescent is the lower border of your lower eyelid muscle (the orbicularis oculi). In younger people, it is barely noticeable. But as many individuals age, especially beyond their 40s, the crescent can become an obvious, unattractive fullness along the upper cheekbone.

A traditional facelift not only fails to address this bulge, but the procedure can actually make it worse **(Figure 3-16)**. By not repositioning the lower eyelid muscle upwards, the surgeon virtually guarantees that if this mound is beginning to appear, it will eventually become worse. Additionally, if the fat under the eye was not preserved, and a hollow eye is also developing, the malar crescent will be even more prominent. Considered together, these two markers are noticeable reminders of cosmetic surgery.

The maneuver I described for remedying the lateral sweep and the hollow eye also eliminates the malar crescent **(Figure 3-17)**. Since the cheek lift elevates the whole muscle mass of the lower eyelid and cheek and secures it to the orbital bone, the results are not only dramatic, but long-lasting **(Figures 3-18 and 3-19)**.

I now see ten-year follow-up patients with a stable high cheek mass **(Figure 3-20)**. If you go through surgery, you deserve a great long-lasting result. You want something worth your time and expense.

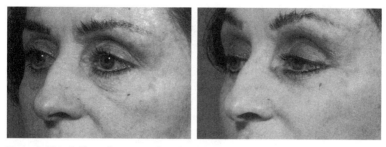

Figure 3-16: Left: The malar crescent (arrow), obvious as a conventional facelift aged. Right, Smooth contour of the upper cheek restored with the Composite.

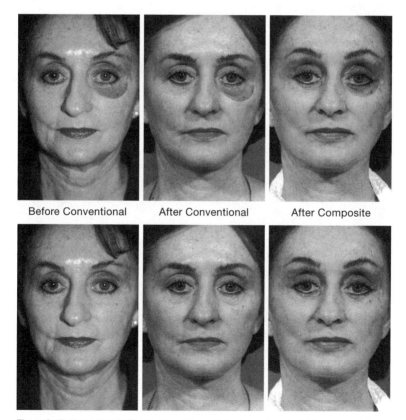

Before Conventional   After Conventional   After Composite

Figure 3-17: Upper photos: The lower eyelid muscle has been drawn in. Note no change in position between "before" and "after" a conventional facelift. Note the improvement after the Composite Facelift.

107

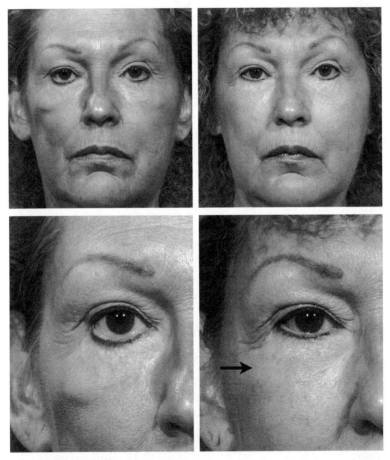

Figure 3-18: Note correction of the pulled-down eye and elimination of the malar crescent (arrow) when the cheek is lifted with the Composite.

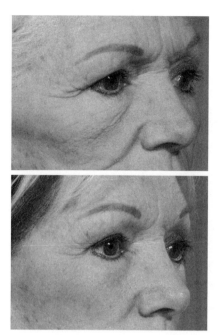

Figure 3-19: Eliminating the malar crescent restores a more youthful contour to the cheek.

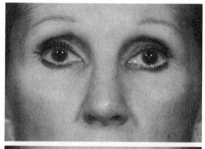

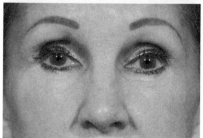

Figure 3-20: Top: After conventional and before Composite procedure. Bottom: Ten years after the Composite, the cheek still appears youthful.

The Anatomy Behind The Cheek Lift

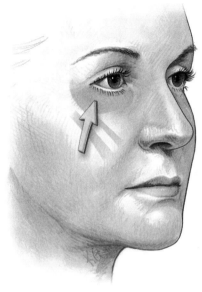

An integral part of the Composite Facelift is the cheek lift, done by using a zygomaticus-orbicularis flap (zygorbicular, for short), a technique that I developed and published in 1998. It is this maneuver that creates the high cheek mass, the look of youth. The fat of your cheek always emphasized in drawings of babies and children as the hallmark of youth and beauty, rides on top of some muscles called the zygomaticus, and is attached to the overlying skin. We cannot sew this fat to anything since it won't hold stitches. But lifting the cheek fat sandwiched between the skin and muscle as one piece (represented by the three-layer arrow in the illustration) and attaching it firmly to the bone on the side of the eye itself gives a stable, high cheek mass. The more effectively the cheek mass is repositioned, the more youthful the face, and the less chance of ever acquiring the signs of having had facelift surgery. The patients in **Figures 3-21 and 3-22** demonstrate the repositioning of the cheek mass to correct a "facelifted" appearance.

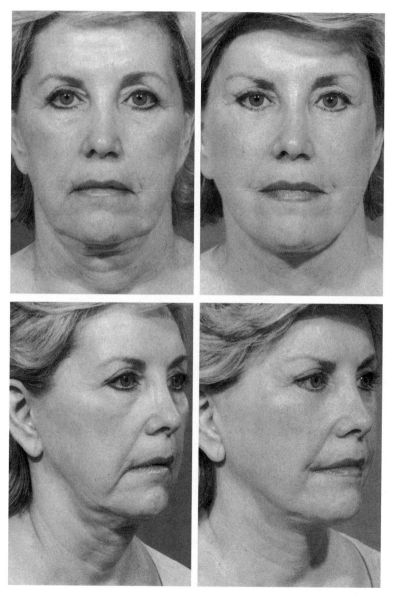

Figure 3-21: Before and after photos show the effect of repositioning the "cheek mass" upward. See her color photos for an illustration of the movement of the cheek fat.

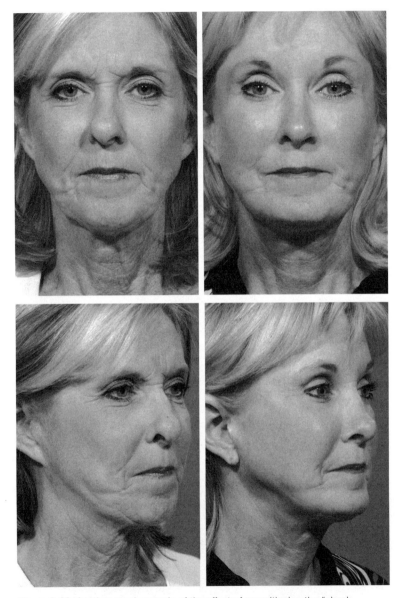

Figure 3-22: Another good example of the effect of repositioning the "cheek mass" upward. A brow lift, chin implant, and rhinoplasty help balance the face. Note earlobe revision.

Other Telltale Signs of Surgery

There are a number of distortions that scream "facelift surgery!" that aren't necessarily the result of the aging of a facelift, but are caused by the technique that was used.

Problem – Earlobe Displacement

Everyone seems to know that it is the ear that often betrays a facelift **(Figures 3-23, 3-24)**. Pulled-down earlobes may happen at the time of the original procedure, or can develop with time. The most dramatic of

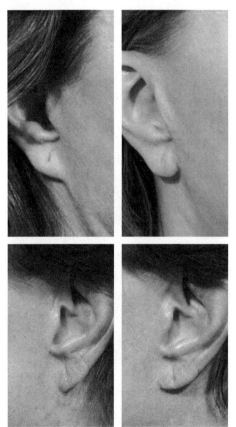

these distortions has been called "the pixie ear." The natural contour of the earlobe can usually be restored, but this is often difficult. The surgeon must use the same facelift incision and recruit more skin from the neck and lower face. It is extremely difficult to correct earlobe problems with a limited operation. In some cases they cannot be corrected fully, as the generous amount of loose skin on the face needed to make these corrections may not be available.

Figure 3-23: Two patients whose earlobes were distorted by a conventional facelift and repaired with the Composite.

Often the earlobe is not distorted, but simply pulled

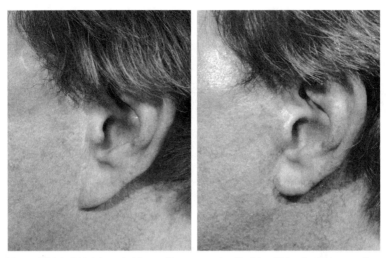

Figure 3-24: Left: Earlobe pulled forward by a conventional incision. Right: Contour restored with the Composite.

forward, another tip-off that a facelift has been done. This can be more noticeable when the earlobe is inherently large. When a patient has a large aging earlobe, I can always reduce the lobe to fit the new younger-looking face.

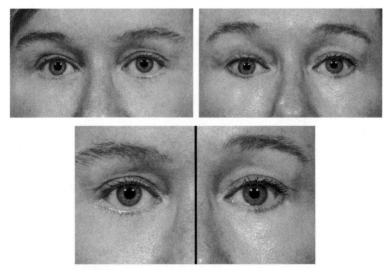

Figure 3-25: Upper left: Several years following a conventional procedure, this patient shows a pulled-down lid. Upper right: Two years after correction of her lower lids. Bottom photo: comparing the left eye before and after revision.

114

Problem – The Pulled Down Eyelid

It is not uncommon to see the lower eyelid pulled down, or to notice a different level when comparing the two eyelids **(Figures 3-25 through 3-27)**. There are several reasons this may occur. The most common is when too much skin or too much fat has been removed, and the lower eyelid reveals too much sclera (white of the eye). This appearance is called "scleral show" and is not only unsightly, but can lead to dryness of the eye, requiring drops and ointment. Anytime a surgeon, even an expert, operates on the lower eyelid, there is a possibility that scleral show can occur. The surgeon must be prepared to correct it—usually not a complicated operation. Many people with "round eyes" inherently have a degree of scleral show before surgery. As always, expectations of the end result of your procedure must be discussed with your surgeon.

Today, a surgeon can control the eyelid level pretty well, but on occasion a more severe scleral show will require a more complicated correction **(Figure 3-28)**. Without question, the eyelid is the most complicated and often least predictable part of facial rejuvenation. It is no wonder that many surgeons who do eyelid surgery infrequently, stay away from this area. A pulled-down eye is very noticeable, more so than any other problem area following facelifts.

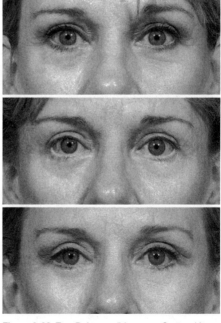

Figure 3-26: Top: Before eyelid surgery. Center: After a conventional procedure elsewhere. Bottom: After septal reset and eyelid revision.

115

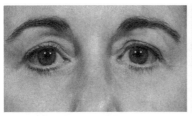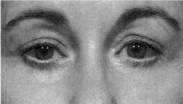

Figure 3-27: Three previous blepharoplasties left this woman with downward sloping eyelid corners. Right: After correction.

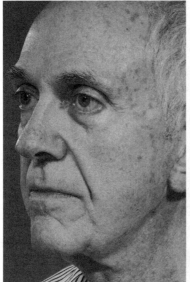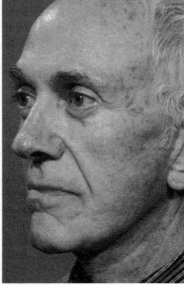

Figure 3-28: Left: This gentleman had facelift and eyelid surgery 13 years previous. Rght: Two years after a secondary Composite Facelift and eyelid correction.

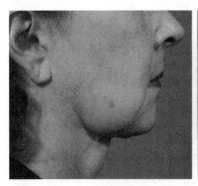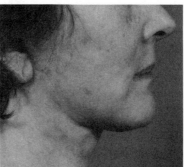

Figure 3-29: Left: Overcorrected neck. Right: Composite revision.

Problem – Post-Op Neck Deformities

The neck is frequently omitted in primary facelifts, or often a more limited neck procedure is done in conjunction with a traditional facelift. Even in the best hands, necks can pose problems following surgery. Because the neck changes appearance with every movement of your body and face, a true evaluation of the static neck is never possible, as it is with eyelids and cheeks. There is a saying that men extend their neck while shaving, so they think they always look young, while women see their neck while looking down in their makeup mirror, and think they always look old. I believe there is some truth to that theory.

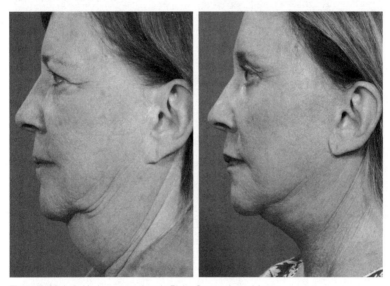

Figure 3-30: Left: Undercorrected neck. Right: Composite revision.

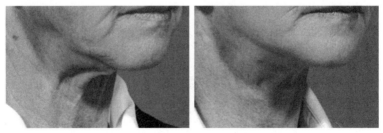

Figure 3-31: Left: "Cords" formed by the platysma muscle. Right: Revised with the Composite Facelift.

117

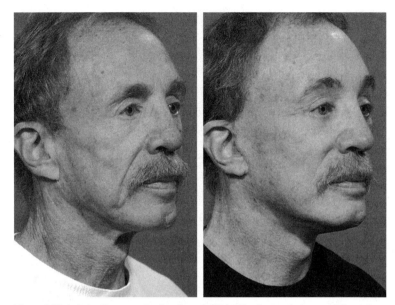

Figure 3-32: Left: Another example of neck cords. Right: The Composite improved the neck, corrected the lateral sweep, and lifted the lower eyelid.

Typically, there may be either too much, not enough, or uneven removal of fat from the neck **(Figure 3-29)**. Excess fat is easier to correct **(Figure 3-30)**. Overly defatted necks are impossible to totally correct. Uneven areas of fat will be seen as abnormal even to the casual observer.

The front edges of the platysma muscle may be visible as unsightly cords or bands **(Figures 3-31, 3-32)**. (The platysma is the muscle that horses use to flick flies off of their skin. It is rudimentary in humans, a leftover of primitive man, and only occurs in the neck.) Cords and excess fat appear normal in the unoperated face, but become very obvious in the facelifted patient when not addressed.

You also need to be aware that the salivary glands located in the neck may be more conspicuous following surgery. The submandibular salivary glands can be felt just under the jawbone. They vary in size depending on what you eat. Removing them may be difficult, and even somewhat risky, since there is an important nerve nearby. Most surgeons prefer to leave them alone.

Problem – Unsightly Incisions

Ideally, all facelift incisions should be placed in areas where they are difficult to see. This is not always possible, but every attempt is made to

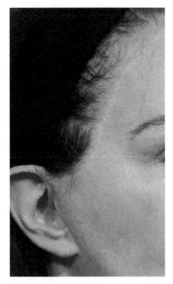

hide telltale scars. Your individual skin type will affect the appearance of healed scars. Often scars are more noticeable because the skin remains a different color, and some skin types heal with some spread to the scar regardless of what surgery is done **(Figure 3-33)**.

The placement of a facelift incision around the ears differs according to the individual surgeon **(Figure 3-34)**. I prefer the incision to curl inside the tragus, the cartilage in front of the opening of the ear. There are surgeons who put

Figure 3-33: Incisions made in front of the hairline are virtually impossible to hide with revision surgery.

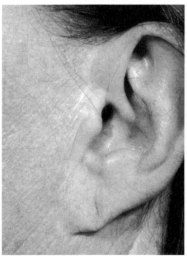
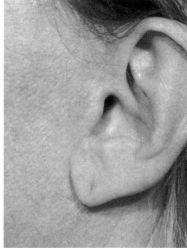

Figure 3-34: These photos show why I prefer to make the incision behind the tragus. Right: The same ear after the Composite revision.

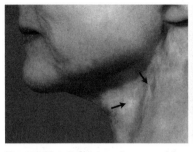 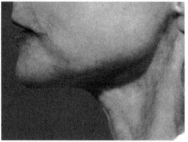

Figure 3-35: Left: Skin loss after surgery left scars on this lady's neck. Right: Some improvement achieved with revision surgery.

the incision in front, thinking it heals better there. I have found that in the event of poor healing, or infection, or too much tension, a scar in front becomes impossible to camouflage, even with makeup.I prefer the incision inside the tragus for men as well. If a scar widens, or if it was placed too far in front of the ear, it can usually be improved when the revision surgery is done.

In some patients there may be wide areas of scarring from skin loss around the ears or neck **(Figure 3-35)**. This was seen more frequently years ago when we didn't know that smokers were at risk for poor healing. We now know that nicotine causes diminished blood flow to the skin. Too much tension, or even pressure from a collection of blood under the skin, can cause wide areas of skin to die if the blood supply is already compromised. While it is impossible to remove all such scarring, improvements can be made, even doing a little bit at a time over a number of months.

The two gentlemen in **Figures 3-36 and 3-37** came to me for help with multiple problems resulting from previous surgery done elsewhere. Note the improvements seen in all areas after their revisions. The pulled-down ear, lateral sweep, and hollow eyes, as well as the downward slant of the lower eyelids have been corrected.

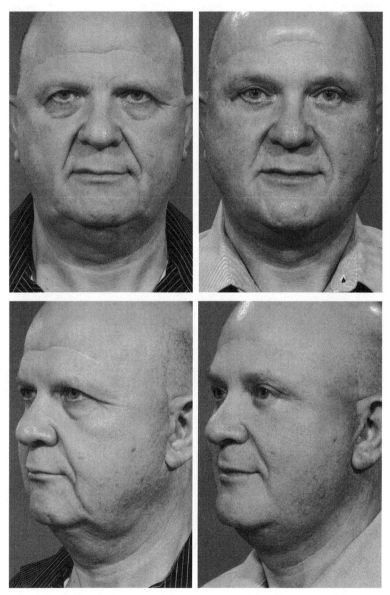

Figure 3-36: Left: Numerous stigmata from previous surgery, including a curious scar from an attempted browlift. Right: All-around improvement with the Composite procedure, including correction of the lateral sweep.

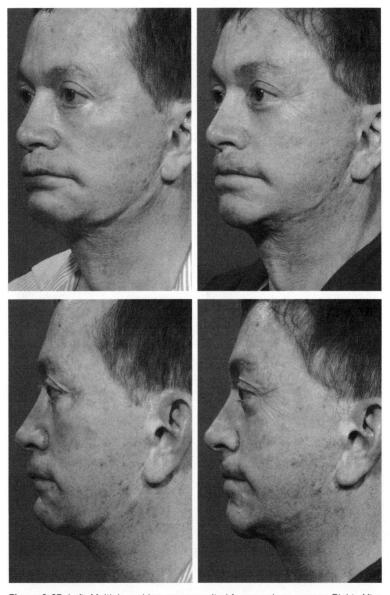

Figure 3-37: Left: Multiple problem areas resulted from previous surgery. Right: After extensive revision, which included correction of the pulled-down lower eyelids, thinning of overly-injected lips, excisions of unevenness of the neck and removal of cheek and chin implants. Tight skin prevented correction of the facelift incision in front of the ear.

Less Is Less, More Is More

Although the lateral sweep, hollow eyes and malar crescent are distinctive spin-offs of a conventional (lateral vector) facelift technique, collectively they are evidence of a face that has lost its youthful glow, and also its youthful harmony. The Composite Facelift can bring back both.

I am concerned about the minimally invasive techniques that have been introduced to nip and tuck younger patients before they start visibly sagging. In fact, many of the newest facial cosmetic surgical approaches have been inspired by patients who are not quite ready for a complete facelift but who want to tweak their looks before they reach 45 or 50.

With procedures like the *Mini Facelift,* (also known as the *Weekend Facelift* or the *S-Lift*), the *Short Scar Lift*, and other minimal approaches, physicians are accommodating people who think they are getting some improvement with a small procedure. The long-term consequences are rarely explained to patients. Remember that your face is a sum of its parts, and doing one part only may lead to disillusionment and disappointment following surgery. Instant gratification is everyone's goal, but it often comes with a price.

> No matter how you look at it, lesser is less and the older you are, that lesser becomes least. More is more, and that means more parts of the face, more longevity, more harmony, more money and more recovery.

Much of the promotion of noninvasive or minimally invasive procedures has been done by the companies that manufacture injectables and energy-based devices, as well as by non-surgeons. There is a national marketing campaign for a "liquid facelift" that uses injectables to fill out parts of the face. This is appealing to many patients, who notice unwanted surgical appearances wherever they go. It is understandable that they are seeking an alternative to surgery. The early results are impressive, and in time this may become the standard for younger people. But while many patients look good, some end up looking bloated from over-filling. At the present time, long-term results are not known for some of these treatments.

Certainly for patients who have noticeable problems following facelift surgery, revision surgery remains the only effective and long-lasting corrective treatment.

The Composite Facelift does more than just improve separate areas of your face. The parts of your face have aged together, and improving them together at the same time can restore the harmony of youth. By eliminating problems from earlier surgery, we can also restore confidence and self-esteem. ❖

Tales from The Operating Room

The best way to illustrate the challenges and emotional upheaval patients may experience when their surgery has had unsatisfactory results is to hear it from the patients themselves. In compiling this book, I asked some of my own patients to relate their personal stories in their own words.

The stories on the following pages are true, but names have been changed.

SHERYL'S STORY

"I was referred to a plastic surgeon in Dallas who was supposed to be very good. I went to him for a facelift and browlift at age 55 because my daughter got married that year, and I wanted my face to look nice in time for the wedding. I was happy at first, but by the time the wedding came around, when I saw the pictures, I started to notice that I was getting sags on the side of my face."

Sheryl had a very common experience. Initial results with SMAS procedures can look good because of the swelling that plumps up the face. But with a traditional facelift, as healing continues and swelling subsides, relaxation can return.

"Nine months after the surgery, I was drooping again. The surgeon told me that everyone is different. He offered to go in and do a string procedure to tighten it up. Then he suggested that Thermage would help and it would last about six months to a year. I didn't want either of those. He told me it was the structure of my face, but I just didn't buy it. He finally admitted that it didn't hold up. I had already paid almost $30,000 and I was upset and I wasn't ready to undergo another seven-hour procedure. I'd had a good feeling about the first surgeon, but that was a mistake. Even my brow was starting to crease in the front after such a short time. I wanted to look around for someone else to correct it. My husband thought I was crazy!"

Thirteen months after her first facelift, Sheryl came to me for revision surgery. I told her that her surgeon was an excellent surgeon—it was the technique that was the problem.

"I found Dr. Hamra and he told me about the Composite Lift and how he does it. He said he could improve on what was already done. This surgery is not for sissies. The whole experience was completely different. Recovery was much longer because of the work he had to do on my

eyes. I couldn't see for two weeks. Although I didn't bruise much, there was a lot more swelling. But I would send anyone to Dr. Hamra. His staff is wonderful and they tell you exactly what to expect. My whole face looks better. It's even and has a much younger look. I would definitely recommend his procedure, even though it was a little tougher than the first one was. My husband is a physician, and he liked my facelift so much that he had one the following year!" ❖

LILLIAN'S STORY

"The first time I had plastic surgery was when I had my eyes done at age 35, and Dr. Hamra did that for me. He did such a wonderful job. My mother and sister had beautiful eyes, but mine were sort of hooded. When I was 45, I went to Dr. Hamra for a facelift, but he told me I was too early and to wait, but I didn't and went to another surgeon who did a facelift on me. I couldn't see the difference. He was a new doctor just starting out..."

As is too often the case, she was disappointed when there was very little change. One must be sure that there is enough aging to justify surgery. Facelifts are not "preventive" operations. They must give an appreciable change to be worth the time and money.

"Fifteen years later I was having breathing problems and went to have it corrected. My nostrils were too small and I couldn't breathe and I snored at night. The surgeon I went to said he could fix it, and while he was there, he could get rid of the bags under my eyes, and offered to do it for free. But I looked like a basset hound after the surgery. I was so depressed. He took out too much skin. My lower lid was pulled down and I looked so bad. I was traumatized. Dr. Hamra was the only one I would go to to fix the problem, and he did."

Surgeons are complimented when a patient returns to them for opinions or corrections.

"I think some day within the next couple of years I'm going to go back to have my face done. I look like a young 60 or maybe late 50s. I don't care so much about my age, and I've earned every wrinkle, but I don't have to show them. Dr. Hamra is a wonderful, caring doctor." ❖

RAINA'S STORY

"I was in the Middle East working as an engineer when a friend under-went cosmetic surgery in Jordan. She had a good result, so I went to see her surgeon. He performed a full facelift with eyelids, and did my nose. After surgery I had difficulty with my left eye. I went back for a second surgery, which wasn't successful. I was in sad shape, and very stressed. I went back to Jordan to have it done a third time, but this time my lower eyelid sagged. He finally recommended that I see Dr. Hamra."

Before coming to me, Raina saw doctors in her hometown on the West Coast. They all had their own theories on how to fix her problems, and there are frequently many good approaches for these difficult cases, but she decided it would be worth the trip to Dallas.

"Dr. Hamra has such great credentials that I decided to go to Texas. I didn't think I could trust anybody else. Dr. Hamra was very professional. He did the surgery to correct what the other surgeon had done, even improving the horrible scars. The man is a magician! There is a huge improvement after his work. He really did a fabulous job. I feel like I am a person again. I can look people in the eyes again. I don't think you can get any better than Dr. Hamra. He is worth his weight in gold." ❖

VIVIAN'S STORY

"You think you do your homework. I am a dentist myself, and the doctor I first went to came with substantial referrals. He was older, not a cowboy, had been around the block, knew how to do things. I had many procedures done at once. I had a facelift, browlift, nose, deep laser resurfacing, and cheek implants. I still have significant scars from the laser. One of my cheek implants was too low, and down far enough to cause numbness in my upper lip. The other one was too high—the top of the implant was too close to my eye."

Multiple procedures can be—and are often best—done at the same time. Resurfacing, however, is an option one can do later. Cheek implants make no sense for the facelift patient, since every Composite Facelift will create a "high cheek mass," using your own tissue to put it back to where it was in youth.

"The whole experience was terrible. The surgeon argued with me, and I was very angry at the way I was treated. I had two facelifts within a year. That surgeon removed the cheek implants, added a chin implant, redid my facelift, and made my eyes look smaller—like little beady eyes. I had to take three weeks off work and was still not ready to go back. I was swollen, bruised, burning and weepy. After the healing was at a point where I didn't have to wear camouflage makeup, I could see that this was not going to be right. Through a series of referrals, I was sent to Dr. Hamra. What a difference! He is very low key and logical. He talked to me about what was there and what I could expect."

Vivian was most concerned about her eyes, but other areas were also not done well. I didn't feel she'd be happy unless I could redo everything.

"Dr. Hamra was right. I wouldn't have been happy just having my eyes redone. I learned a lot from this. Word-of-mouth is the most important

thing. It doesn't matter how much training and experience a surgeon has if they don't have any skills. They can be trained and do the same thing for 25 years and still not do it well. My husband wasn't really supportive—the unsaid "I told you so" was always there. Then there's the money thing—and there's the money thing twice if you have to have the surgery redone. I refer all my patients to Dr. Hamra now." ❖

SYDELL'S STORY

"I had a facelift and my eyes done before, so when I was considering another one, I thought I knew what I wanted. I asked my primary care doctor for some plastic surgeon referrals, and I talked to them, but they weren't telling me what I wanted to hear. The sixth plastic surgeon suggested I see Dr. Hamra."

Sydell recognized that she didn't want the same procedure done again. She had been happy with the initial results, but wasn't pleased with the way her facelift aged.

"Dr. Hamra explained his technique and I understood it. He showed me pictures and that was exactly what I wanted. I didn't think I needed anything pulled back again — it seemed to me that it should go up, not out or to the side. He was the only one I found who was doing that type of operation. If I hadn't found Dr. Hamra, I would still be looking — I didn't want to be pulled back the way I was before. After a number of years, your face starts to droop. I had gone to plastic surgeons and I would say that they ought to go up this way instead of out that way. One surgeon wanted to put in cheek implants to pull it up, but I didn't want cheek implants. I had so many different opinions — and these were all highly thought-of surgeons. I was just going from one to another — they had the right credentials, but they all had their own procedure. I waited eight years after my first facelift to have my face and brow done."

More and more cosmetic surgeons are realizing the importance of vertical repositioning of the face. In particular, moving the tissues of the cheek upwards restores a smooth, youthful contour without the use of cheek implants, which can create a wide, angular look to the face.

"You don't see the pulling back towards your ear. I see some ladies and I say to myself that they should see Dr. Hamra! It is so obvious to me now."

Since she had already undergone a conventional facelift, Sydell could compare the difference in recovery time between traditional procedures and the Composite Facelift.

"After surgery, it takes awhile before you can look at yourself and realize that the result is what you wanted! But now I get amazing reactions. I am 71 years old and when I tell people that, no one believes me. I say, "Would I say I am 71 years old if I'm not?" If I knew anyone who was considering a facelift, I most certainly would send them to Dr. Hamra. He doesn't make you feel like he is an elitist — he's just so nice. I could not be more satisfied. Dr. Hamra is my hero — I love him!" ❖

RITA'S STORY

"Dr. Hamra changed my life. I had previous surgery in Chicago with a doctor who was very well thought-of, but it was a catastrophe. Before my surgery, I checked on lawsuits and he had none on his record."

Rita was smart to try to research the doctor, but discovered that whether or not a doctor has been sued can be irrelevant, as good surgeons can have frivolous lawsuits and unqualified surgeons may never have one.

"I looked the same or older after the surgery. I lost too much skin behind my ears. My left eye had scleral show. The surgeon also did fat injections. I had eight hours of surgery, and then he bandaged me up in a way that ruined the neck. I looked horrible."

Rita had skin loss because too much tension was placed on the skin, which compromised the blood supply.

"No one in Chicago would touch me. They said I could not have surgery for ten years and my neck was ruined. The Chief of Plastic Surgery at the medical school was following my wound healing because I had gaping wounds. I had scar tissue there and horrible white areas. I looked like I was a burn victim. My neck was so tight, I couldn't even move it. Finally I was referred to Dr. Hamra, and 11 months later he redid my surgery. When I went to see him, I expected him to say no. Instead he said, "no problem." He has an optimistic attitude and it passes to the patient. I felt very confident with him. I was fortunate enough to find him and I don't know what I would have done without him."

Frequently one must wait a year to re-operate in order to allow the scar tissue to soften and mature.

"I am still suffering from the consequences of my first procedure with the Chicago surgeon, which impacted my nerve endings and, in fact,

I no longer practice law because of a loss of stamina. However, in terms in my looks, I never looked better — thanks to Dr. Hamra. I am 65, and I look 50. My facelift is perfect and it doesn't look like a facelift. It looks very natural. I will always be grateful to Dr. Hamra." ❖

STACY'S STORY

"When I was referred to the first plastic surgeon, I had not seen any of his work, which was stupid on my part."

It's wise to read about facelifts before interviewing a plastic surgeon, so you will be able to ask intelligent questions about his technique. Don't be afraid to ask to see photographs.

"I was young then. I am 75 now and people think that I am in my 50s. My first surgeon created lumps under the skin under my eye area. When he lifted the face up, he didn't put it back right. I am a perfectionist. I lived with it for a long time. I had naturally almond eyes and he rounded them so they looked strange. I waited about 10 years before I had my second procedure. I went to Dr. Hamra because I had heard of him from people who had wonderful face and eye lifts. One of my girlfriends had gone to him, and she looked great and still does. He took one look at me and said, "You look pretty but you can look prettier." Dr. Hamra's technique lifts upwards instead of pulling to the side and making it look like you've had surgery. With the first doctor, it looked like I had surgery. And when you pull to the side it drops faster than when you pull it up. Dr. Hamra's Composite Facelift lifts in a vertical direction so my eyes and cheeks were corrected. I had hardly any bruising. He did my face, neck and eyes and got rid of the lumps. After my hospital stay, I felt good enough to join family members for a Thanksgiving celebration in my home."

Everyone responds differently to surgery. Stacy had an easy recovery!

"Dr. Hamra is a very positive kind of surgeon. He has confidence and has that air about him. He is very into you — he knows what you want and he does it. He is smart and artistic, too. His mannerisms are polished and classy. The other surgeon had come in jeans and a t-shirt at

times. Dr. Hamra is always personable and well-groomed — and that's important to me. After surgery, he has a no-nonsense way about him. He reassures you every step, and kind of makes you feel like you're someone special. He makes you feel that if something happens, he'll take care of it." ❖

CAROLINE'S STORY

"I just think Dr. Hamra is best doctor in the world! One of my friends in Florida had a facelift done by him and I said that if ever I had a facelift, he would be my man. She looked better than any of my other friends who'd had facelifts. I think he took 20 years off her. So when it was time, I went to see him. The whole surgery went just wonderfully, though it took a while to look really good, because of the swelling. He did a facelift and my brows and eyelids. He has gone back and done more to my eyes since then."

Sometimes a touch-up is desired for the optimal look, and can often be done as an office procedure.

"I stayed one night in the hospital and had very good care. Dr. Hamra's staff was just wonderful and they called to check on me every day."

I keep everyone in the hospital the first night, but many patients ask to stay longer.

"The result made me look 10 years younger; I am 67 and I look like I am 57. My friends think it looks good and natural. One of my friends had a facelift done by someone else, and wasn't satisfied at all. She has the kind of skin that wrinkles really easily. Her mother was very wrinkly too and she inherited it from her. The laugh lines at the corners of her eyes are still very deep. My eyes are smooth and my cheeks are smooth, too. Dr. Hamra did a wonderful job. His technique is the best. Instead of going behind your ears and lifting it to the sides, he lifts it up towards your eyes. I think it makes it look more natural. You see faces that really look like plastic, but I look really good!" ❖

FOR SECOND-TIME PATIENTS:
10 Questions to Ask Your Surgeon

1. If you use the SMAS procedure to correct me, what parts of my face will you include? Will it correct my lateral sweep?

2. What parts of my face are excluded? If you don't do the forehead lift, will it then match the face?

3. How do you handle my hollow lower eyelids? Can you do a septal reset? If you use an injectable filler, how long will it last, and how much will I have to pay for touch-up injections in the future?

4. How long can I expect a corrective procedure to last?

5. If you correct my facelift and do not use a Composite Lift, what procedure will you use, and can you assure me it will work?

6. Will you do a forehead lift and if so, can you prevent my high forehead from going higher?

7. How do you correct that windswept look?

8. Can you get the incisions to go from outside to inside the ear cartilage?

9. Can you make my malar crescent disappear?

10. Do I need a peel or laser procedure to improve my skin?

PART FOUR

FINDING THE RIGHT SURGEON

The most important part
of having a great facelift
is finding the right surgeon,
who is using the right technique.

Now that you know what kind of facelift will give you the long-lasting, natural results that you want, you are ready for the next step: identifying the right surgeon for your facelift. There are many competent cosmetic surgeons practicing today, but finding one who does the Composite procedure will take time and research. Perhaps you have already identified a physician with whom you are comfortable, someone who communicates well and has earned your trust. But you still want to make sure that this person is familiar with the methods discussed in the previous chapters, and can perform them adeptly on you. Whether you're a first-time candidate or repeat patient, the following pages will help you make important decisions about your new face.

If you're looking for a corrective facelift, you may be wondering if you should you go back to the surgeon who did the original procedure. That is a very reasonable question, since it is easy to fault your doctor when a facelift fails. Who better to blame for the tension and pulls across your cheeks and jawline than the physician who did your initial work? But as I have explained, it is usually the technique, not the surgeon, that is the real problem.

If it has been several years since your first surgery, your surgeon may have learned the newer procedures. The vast majority of plastic surgery specialists are well prepared to do what their patients need and want. They have worked for many years to solidify their knowledge of the underlying anatomy that provides function and gives every face its unique features and beauty.

You must be very selective, especially if you are looking for someone who is adept at performing facelifts that will leave a lasting, stunning result. All of the general advice that applies to selecting a cosmetic surgeon in the first place applies here. You want a specialist schooled in the broader field of plastic surgery with the right board-certified skills and long-term experience to do your facial rejuvenation. Beyond prioritizing facelifts in their practice, this person should also have a track record with the Composite technique. How do you find this special mix of skills, training and competence? It's not magic. It just takes commitment to doing the research.

Qualifications Are Paramount

If you've already had a facelift, you know all about tapping your friends, family members and even your physician to find a quality surgeon. Even if you are doing this for the first time, you're probably aware that approaching people you trust for names of surgeons can yield a bevy of great recommendations worth a closer look. But identifying someone comfortable with advanced procedures like the Composite procedure requires even more attention to detail. You will need to scrutinize the qualifications of your best candidates very carefully, especially if this is your second time around.

You should consider the following in your search:

Education, Training, Board Certification

The first item on your agenda is to make sure that your surgeon is actually trained in plastic surgery. You may be asking, "Don't all physicians who do facial operations have that background?" In a word, no. Many doctors marketing their facial rejuvenation skills these days come from various other specialties, such as dermatology and oral surgery.

Granted, they may have one or two years of additional training to perform facial procedures along with their first specialty. But they do not undergo the same five- or six-year plastic surgery residency that surgeons devoted to this field take on to fine-tune their reconstructive and cosmetic skills.

To demonstrate what an aesthetic surgeon brings to the table, just consider that after medical school, he or she spends three to five years in general surgery or otolaryngology with an additional two to three years focused on plastic surgery. Plastic surgeons receive training primarily in reconstructive procedures—those medically necessary techniques used to restore the function or appearance of a damaged structure. Repairing a cleft palate or a facial injury falls in this arena. But they're also exposed to cosmetic surgery—the elective procedures, like standard facelifts, nasal surgery and body contouring done purely to improve otherwise normal features. Eventually most doctors focus on one of those broad plastic surgery areas, becoming proficient in a wide range of procedures or maybe just one.

In either case, by the time a new aesthetic surgeon is established, he or she has spent many hours mastering plastic surgery skills under the tutelage of many others. Some physicians polish their abilities through post-residency fellowships with a physician or in a hospital program. But the real fine-tuning for cosmetic surgeons comes over the next years as they build their experience and reputations for very good work. Throughout that time, they are constantly engaged in continuing education. Although updating your skills is a requirement in medicine, good cosmetic surgeons want to do it routinely to perform the best procedures they can.

Board certification means that your surgeon has jumped through additional rigorous credentialing hoops put in place by a medical specialty to demonstrate competence. Although it is voluntary, it indicates that your doctor has completed an accredited residency program and passed a series of required oral and written exams.

But not every board will do. You're looking for evidence that your surgeon is a "diplomate" (or "candidate" if their status is pending) of the American Board of Plastic Surgery (ABPS), a panel focused solely on certifying doctors trained in this field. ABPS is the only plastic surgery organization recognized by the American Board of Medical Specialties (ABMS), the umbrella agency for more than 20 specialty-accrediting boards. Of course, you can find a qualified cosmetic surgeon who is not board certified. But by having the ABPS seal of approval, physicians demonstrate that they're committed enough to quality clinical outcomes and patient safety to be evaluated by their peers. They also show that they are willing to engage in continuing education. Since certifications are usually renewed every 10 years, you will also want to see if this surgeon's status is up-to-date at **www.abms.org**.

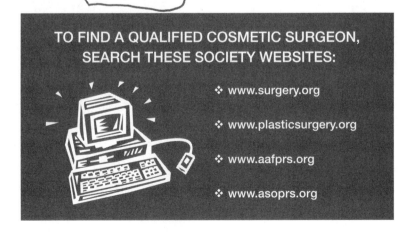

TO FIND A QUALIFIED COSMETIC SURGEON, SEARCH THESE SOCIETY WEBSITES:

❖ www.surgery.org

❖ www.plasticsurgery.org

❖ www.aafprs.org

❖ www.asoprs.org

It is preferable that your surgeon be board-certified in plastic surgery because you want someone who has learned as much about reconfiguring the human face and body as possible to handle the unique conditions of each patient. ABPS diplomates have demonstrated proficiency in a full spectrum of cosmetic and reconstructive procedures. They are ready, in terms of their knowledge and preparation, to take on your face.

There are two other specialties that have highly qualified surgeons I respect. Ophthalmic plastic surgeons are ophthalmologists who have advanced training in plastic and reconstructive surgery of the eyelids. They are the doctors that many of us depend on when eyelid problems are seen following surgery. Plastic surgeons doing advanced techniques usually maintain a strong and respectful relationship with these surgeons. There are also the facial plastic surgeons, who are ENT (ear, nose, and throat) surgeons with advanced training. There are many surgeons from this specialty who I respect as well, as some of the most significant advances in rhinoplasty surgery have come from this group of surgeons.

No Substitute for Experience

Board certification is certainly an indicator of a physician's readiness to perform plastic surgery. But experience trumps everything, especially if the goal is to correct the ills of a past procedure with a new approach! You really want someone who has proven his or her skills with conventional procedures before taking on the Composite technique. Why is that important? To be adept at an advanced procedure, the surgeon should first be comfortable moving your facial tissue with basic approaches. The number of procedures performed per month is not essential unless it shows that the doctor puts other cosmetic or reconstructive surgeries over facelifts.

The bigger key is that the surgeon you choose knows and has experience with new advanced techniques like the Composite Facelift. Since the learning curve for this approach is steep, not everyone who generates beautiful results with traditional facelifts will be interested in performing its sophisticated maneuvers. In fact, most aesthetic surgeons still do the SMAS procedure exclusively, in large part because they're comfortable with it and in general the results are acceptable. The problem arises if you need a correction. By undergoing the same technique that caused the distortions in the first place, you put yourself at risk for even more problems in the future.

An aesthetic surgeon who can perform a Composite Facelift or similar procedure will be able to demonstrate that he or she has an entirely different plan. This surgeon not only can talk about rejuvenating the entire face in one integrated surgery, but can also offer a viable solution when you ask the hard questions:

❖ How will you fix the pull in my face or prevent it in the future?

❖ How will you correct my eyes so they don't appear hollow down the road?

❖ How will you deal with the pooches on my cheekbones?

The surgeon should be able to say that your cheek muscle and fat will be lifted vertically to eliminate future pulling. Regarding the stigmata connected to your eye, the under-eye muscle and remaining fat will be repositioned over your orbital bone to restore the smooth eye-to-cheek contours. Of course there will be other things to cover, but the point is to find someone who can show you that they have the experience, understand the complexities of the Composite Facelift, and are up to the task — or can offer a similar technique that will correct the unacceptable appearance that bothers you.

Many patients ask if the doctor has to be an artist to produce great, long-lasting results. Yes and no. Once an operation is standardized, the surgeon must be a good craftsman to reproduce again and again a really good result. Sensitivity to aesthetics is obviously important for a stunning outcome. Every cosmetic surgeon must have a sense of symmetry and proportion to create a youthful look. But as we have learned, rejuvenating your face is actually more about technique than artistry. Standard facelift approaches can hamstring any good surgeon in their attempts to achieve a long-lasting, harmonious result. With the Composite approach those same surgeons can create an enduring work of art.

Complementary Procedures

When seeing many patients for either a first or second time facelift, I am never surprised to find that they have also previously undergone other cosmetic procedures. The type of patient who is considering a facelift is often likely to have sought improvement through surgery on other areas of his or her face and/or body in the past. As the awareness of cosmetic surgery for the face and body has increased over the past few decades, I do see more patients who started years ago having cosmetic surgical procedures. Although the primary or secondary patients I see are generally considering facelift surgery, many request information concerning either primary or secondary surgery of their nose, breasts, and body as well. Combining certain procedures — for example, a nasal revision with a facelift procedure — is quite common and deemed safe in most otherwise healthy patients. In some cases, we are also able to combine a breast lift, breast augmentation, tummy tuck, or liposuction with a facelift operation, depending on many factors, including the surgical facility, the health of the patient, the available after-care, and the judgment of the surgeon.

Nasal Surgery

There have been enormous changes in the approach to reshaping the nose in the last three decades, as compared to previous periods when rhinoplasty was considered a simple technique. In most cases, rhinoplasty operations done many years ago utilized a "closed" approach, meaning that the surgeon made most of the anatomical changes inside the nose working almost blindly. Thus it is not uncommon to find patients who are unhappy with their nose because it was either made too small, or they have developed deformities of the cartilage and bones as time went by. Today, with the ability to perform "open" rhinoplasty, surgeons can more easily and completely re-examine nasal procedures done in the past.

Patients undergoing a facelift procedure can take the opportunity to address a previous rhinoplasty that may have caused some disappointment over the years. In the case of a patient undergoing either a primary or secondary facelift, a secondary rhinoplasty offers a good chance of improvement over a previous suboptimal result. Newer techniques incorporate the addition of cartilage grafts taken from the patient's nose or behind the ear to restore areas where the cartilage was too aggressively removed.

Open procedures can benefit the mature first-time rhinoplasty patient as well. We can actually use techniques that prevent the nose from looking too small and create a shape that is much more complimentary.

Breast Surgery

Often breast procedures are done at the same time as a primary or secondary facelift. The patient may simply have the desire to make her breasts larger with breast implants, which consist of a silicone shell filled with either saline or silicone gel. Mature patients who have always had small breasts are still good candidates for breast augmentation, just as they would have been in their younger years. Women with excess skin or relaxation of the breasts may want either a simple breast lift to reshape the breast without an implant, or have implants placed as well for enhanced volume.

Breast reduction surgery is also commonly requested. The incisions for the breast lift and breast reduction are similar; an incision is typically made around the areola and extended vertically to a horizontal incision at the crease under the breast. These scars tend to heal very well over time and the results have excellent longevity.

Another commonly requested procedure is breast revision surgery. It is well known that one of the most common complications of breast implants is scar tissue formation. The implant itself does not change, but rather scar tissue develops around the implant and creates an unwanted look and feel of firmness. It is a rather simple procedure to remove the old breast implant, release the scar tissue within the pocket, and then replace the implant with an updated model.

Body Contouring

Body contouring today has become much more advanced due to improvements in techniques and in technology. Women (and some men) who start with ideal silhouettes will usually age well if they look after themselves—except for the abdominal area. Loose skin and abdominal muscle separation can become a problem even for those who were always well built, and particularly for women after childbirth. On occasion, additional layers of abdominal fat may have also developed. All three of these problems can be addressed by skin removal, muscle repair and fat removal.

Liposuction is almost always successful for removing excess fat from the thighs ("saddlebags") but may not be effective in the abdominal area when the patient's age means the skin will not shrink after liposuction as it does in younger people. Liposuction only deals with fat. There may be excess skin and muscle looseness due to multiple childbirths and weight fluctuations, which also need to be addressed. The most disappointing result following simple liposuction is when the fat is removed but the skin does not shrink nicely. An abdominoplasty, or tummy tuck, can remove excess skin as well as fat, and tighten up loose muscles. For the facelift patient desiring body contouring, an evaluation would be necessary to see if a combination of a tummy tuck and hip and thigh liposuction might be the best approach. Today's procedures can be very effective and offer long-lasting results.

On the other hand, I also frequently see patients who have had liposuction or abdominoplasty with ultimately disappointing results. These situations are easy to improve with revision surgery. Modern abdominoplasty techniques can remarkably transform surgical results that may have been acceptable many years ago, but have become less attractive over time.

An Integrated Approach

The harmony we strive for in facelift surgery is achieved with the Composite Lift because *all portions* of the aging face are repositioned to their youthful positions. Using the same philosophy, many patients, desiring even more, would like to have a younger-shaped body to be "in sync" with their rejuvenated face. Such harmony between the face and body can be achieved with rejuvenation obtained by body contouring procedures. This can be done at the same time, thereby using the same recovery time for both areas, and saving the hospital cost of two separate procedures.

Both face and body procedures are commonly performed by most experienced plastic surgeons. Note that surgeons who specialize only in facial surgery — ENT and ophthalmic surgeons — do not perform surgery of the body, since they do not have the required background in general surgery.

Another important consideration is whether procedures should be combined. Naturally you should discuss this with your surgeon, and their decision will be determined by where they operate and if they feel that these combinations are safe in your case.

One of the real pleasures of the practice of plastic surgery is in seeing a patient who, over the years, has had both body contouring and facial rejuvenation. While diet and exercise promote health and longevity, it is no secret that our outward appearance will inevitably change over time. I have seen patients striving to maintain their youth spend as much annually on a personal trainer as they would spend on a body contouring procedure. *Exercise can have a terrific impact on cardiovascular function, strength, and muscle tone, but it does little or nothing to improve the quality of the skin or reduce sagging and wrinkles.*

Your Consultation

The initial appointment with your surgeon is crucial. If you have had previous facial rejuvenation surgery, you'll have a slightly different agenda than if you're a first-time patient. In both cases, however, you want to make sure that the surgeon sees the same challenges in your face that you see and can correct them to your long-term satisfaction.

Your goal is simple: make sure the surgeon can correct or prevent the "facelifted" look on you!

Be honest in your assessment about your current look. Perhaps your cheeks are sagging when they should still be attractively taut? Or maybe you look gaunt and tired when you were promised a lasting youthful glow? Now that you know the inherent shortcomings of traditional facelifts, and have learned about a different approach, you are ready to talk frankly about what the doctor can do for you. Whatever challenges you see during the discussion, your goal is simple: make sure the surgeon can correct or prevent the "facelifted" look on you!

Medical History and Physical Exam

Since a Composite Facelift is major surgery, and major surgery can put stress on the body, your doctor will assess every aspect of your medical history. Whether this is your first or a subsequent facelift, you'll need to review the issues that may cause complications or compromise your recovery.

Your surgeon will be particularly interested, for instance, in chronic problems such as heart disease, diabetes, and high blood pressure, which can cause problems with the blood supply to the skin and influence how you respond to anesthesia. Similarly, since excessive bleeding, clotting, or other blood disorders can impact healing, you will be asked about your personal and family history with these issues. You may also be asked about other medical problems, such as asthma, allergies and respiratory issues that could affect your recovery.

Since some of the same medications (prescription or over-the-counter) that are safe and effective under normal circumstances can be dangerous when paired with surgery, you'll need to discuss them with your doctor. These include certain blood thinners, pain relievers, and even dietary supplements and herbal remedies. Such preparations as aspirin, ibuprofen, warfarin (Coumadin) and even vitamin E can interfere with clotting and intensify bruising. Your doctor needs to know everything you have been taking.

Because of the effect of nicotine on the skin's blood supply, smoking can cause post-operative skin loss, which produces significant scarring. Smokers must stop weeks ahead of surgery and not start again until weeks later to reduce the chance of complications.

Whether you're undergoing a facelift as a first-time pick-me-up or a second-time correction, just remember that you'll have to have your health issues in order before taking this plunge.

Your surgeon will do a quick examination of your facial structure and skin tone to make certain he or she can obtain an appreciable improvement with the Composite Facelift. After assessing your unique features and issues, the doctor may also suggest additional procedures as a further enhancement. A chin implant, for example, can improve the contour of your neckline significantly.

One of the most important things for your surgeon to know is the health of your eyes and if you have "dry eyes." This condition may alter the procedure in some way. Everyone goes through a period after surgery needing lubricating drops and ointments to keep the corneas moist. Your doctor will want you to be as comfortable as possible during your recovery.

Financial Considerations

Facelifts are generally not covered by insurance. Therefore, a facelift correction, like the initial procedure, will likely require you to pay out-of-pocket costs. Although most surgeons include small touch-ups in their original fees, correcting the face with an entirely new procedure is an entirely new deal. You may be faced with footing the same three costs — for the surgeon, anesthesiologist, and facility — involved in your initial procedure.

Given the extensive nature of a Composite approach, you can anticipate your total expense to probably be higher than a traditional lift. Since fees vary from state to state, how much will depend on the surgeon and the locale. If a subsequent touch-up is done, which is possible with every surgery, you will be responsible for the cost of the anesthesia and surgical facility, but there should never be another fee for the surgeon.

Good facelift surgery does not come cheap, and you must be willing to spend many thousands of dollars for a first-time or follow-up procedure performed by a skilled surgeon. But when you weigh the bottom-line costs against the potential benefits of preventing or correcting a disappointing result, you will discover enormous physical and emotional returns on your investment.

Intuition and the Intangibles — Trust your gut

Once you have done the research and met the surgeon, there is one important step left: Trust your gut. Of course, you want to have a good feeling about the office. Were your questions answered and was everyone attentive to your needs? But your real focus is on the surgeon. Beyond the obvious skills and credentials, you need to be confident that this doctor has an option that's durable over time. Does this person's technique have lasting value? If the answer is "yes," you've likely struck gold! That will only happen if you have done your homework and can ask the right questions.

My Final Thoughts on Facelifting

Facial rejuvenation is not a totally predictable science. Your age, bone structure, skin texture, and overall health and ability to heal will impact how you look in the immediate future. Your surgeon's technique, however, can definitely help you in the long-term. A good cosmetic surgeon, trained in the Composite Facelift, can correct the flaws of a previous surgery or create a stable profile right from the start. There are other approaches, but armed with the knowledge in this book, you should be able to ask the pertinent questions. With a little work, you will find one talented surgeon who can do just that for you. ❖

Glossary

American Board of Medical Specialties (ABMS): The organization that oversees and approves the various specialties and determines the qualifications of those doctors who practice that specialty. www.abms.org

Abdominoplasty: An operation that reshapes the abdomen and is mostly used after pregnancies and after weight loss. Excess skin and fat are removed, and the muscles are usually repaired.

Arcus marginalis release: The arcus marginalis is an anatomical border between the bone of the lower orbit and the tissue that covers the orbital fat. The "release" means to make a cut across this junction to free the fat of the lower eyelid.

Blepharoplasty: An operation of the eyelids, either the upper eyelid or lower eyelid. It does not specify what is done, as there are many blepharoplasty techniques.

BOTOX®: BOTOX® is the brand name of botulinum toxin type A, as marketed by Allergan. This is a drug that temporarily paralyzes muscles. It is most popular for paralyzing the forehead frown muscles, but has numerous uses. The effect usually lasts about three to four months. There are other variations of botulinum toxin type A currently under FDA investigation; DYSPORT® is one that was recently approved.

Browlift: Another term for lifting the brows, whether partly or the complete forehead. It is used interchangeably with forehead lift.

Canthus: The corner of the eye. The lateral canthus is the one further from the nose. The medial canthus is the one near the nose. This

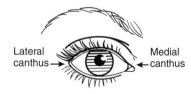

junction joins the upper and lower eyelids and has strong ligaments underneath the skin attaching the canthus to the bones.

Cheek mass: This refers to the cheek fat but more importantly to the highlighted area that can be elevated during a facelift technique which includes the fat with the overlying skin.

Composite Facelift: A Composite Facelift must include several unique features. The most important is the direction of the lift, which features the middle of the face moving toward the eye rather than toward the ear. It always includes the treatment of lower eyelid fat using a septal reset.

Conventional or traditional facelift: These words usually mean that the facelift is a "lateral vector" facelift, meaning the lift is in one direction towards the ear. SMAS lifts, skin lifts, and deep plane lifts are considered conventional procedures.

Coronal: In lifting the forehead, a coronal incision is one that goes over the top of the head from ear to ear. This is to be differentiated from a hairline incision for forehead lifting, which starts from ear to ear but curves forward to run along the hairline of the forehead. The hairline incision will automatically lower a hairline and make the forehead more narrow, where a coronal incision (as well as an endoscopic approach) usually elevates the hairline.

Corrugator muscles: The corrugators are the pair of muscles right above the nose that are responsible for the vertical frown lines

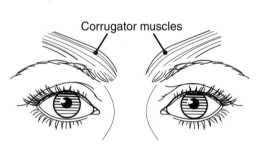

Corrugator muscles

between the eyebrows, giving the face a concerned or "closed look." (Compare with frontalis muscles.) They can be removed during a browlift procedure, or temporarily paralyzed with BOTOX® injections.

Deep Plane Facelift: A facelift where the fat of the cheek as well as the muscle of the lower face is moved toward the ear. It is a lateral vector facelift.

Diplomate: A physician who has been certified by a specialty board after passing the exam for his specialization.

Edema: The accumulation of fluid in the tissues that occurs after surgery that is usually reabsorbed by the body, in varying lengths of time. Edema can also occur in non-surgical situations as in trauma and various diseases.

Endoscopic: An endoscope is an instrument that allows a physician to enter the skin through a small opening to visualize various anatomical areas. It can be used for abdominal and joint surgery, and has been used for browlift procedures and various facelift techniques.

ENT: An expression used to denote the area of medicine specializing in the ear, nose, and throat. This specialty is more formally called otorhinolaryngology.

Festoon: A crescent-shaped outline of the orbicularis oculi muscle that resides on the cheek and is very obvious when the muscle is very excessive.

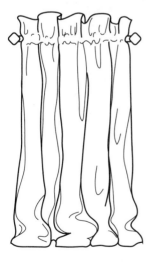
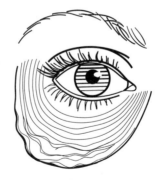

Just as long drapes will pool on the floor, excessive orbicularis oculi muscle can bunch up on the cheek, causing *festoons.*

Frontalis muscle:
A wide muscle of
the forehead that
is responsible for lift-
ing the forehead in
an upward fashion,
causing horizontal
lines on the fore-
head. This muscle
is responsible for

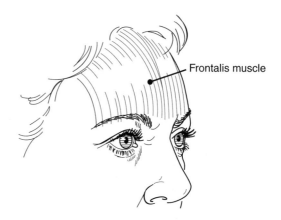

giving the patient the "opened" look or friendly appearance.

Genioplasty: A surgical procedure of the chin involving the chin bone or
simply placement of a chin implant.

Hollow eye: The
concave appear-
ance of the lower
eye area that results
from lack of fat be-
neath the skin. This
can occur normally,
but is commonly

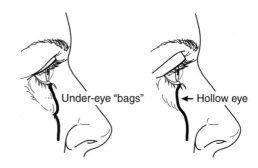

seen following conventional blepharoplasty, when too much fat has been
removed from the lower eyelid and a concave appearance results.

Hyaluronic Acid: A popular choice of temporary filler for facial augmentation. It is a safe substance that gets injected into facial lines and furrows
and attracts water to act as a filling agent. Products available in the US include Restylane®, Perlane®, Juvéderm®, Evolence® and others.

Implant: Any sort of synthetic device that is placed in the body. Breast implants are filled with silicone gel or saline; chin implants can be fashioned
from different materials, such as Gortex®. In the broadest sense, "implant"

can also be applied to the patient's own tissue, such as fat being transferred to a different area of the body.

Injectable: An expression currently used when referring to newer substances that can be injected into the skin to "pump up" areas or lines of the face.

Laser: In plastic surgery, a laser is often used for cutting, taking the place of a scalpel. In recent years, lasers have also been used for various types of skin treatments, including hair removal, acne scars, photorejuvenation, hyperpigmentation and birthmarks.

Lateral sweep: A term applied to the "facelifted" appearance that can result when the lower part of the face is pulled back toward the ear. It is created when the upper parts of the cheeks and face that were not moved or repositioned properly fall down over the tightened lower face and jawline.

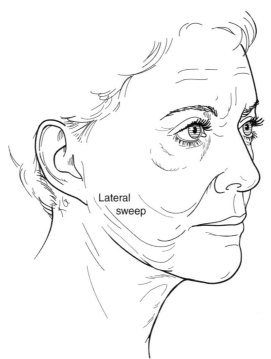

Lateral vector facelift: A lateral vector facelift is a broad classification of facelifts that are more traditional — more conventional — in nature. The direction of the lift of the face is only back toward the ear, as opposed to more modern facelifts that move the lower face toward the ear and the mid-face (cheek area) upwards toward the eye.

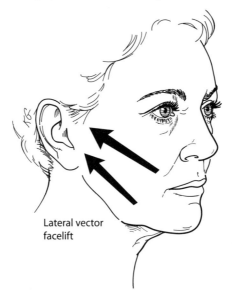

Lateral vector
facelift

Liposuction: A technique of fat removal that was perfected approximately 30 years ago. The fat of various parts of the body or face can be removed or reduced. It is particularly effective with younger patients, as the skin must shrink after liposuction is done to achieve the best result.

Liquid facelift: This is a newer phrase that refers to injection of materials for facial rejuvenation rather than a surgical intervention.

Malar crescent: This is the bottom portion of the lower eyelid muscle (orbicularis oculi) that rests at the junction of the lower eyelid and the cheek. It is normal anatomy, more pronounced in some individuals than others, and may become more obvious with aging or after some facelift techniques.

Malar fat: This is the fat between the junction of the lower eyelid and the nasolabial crease. This is also called the cheek fat, and gives prominence and thus a youthful appearance when in the right position.

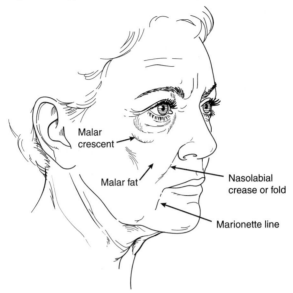

Marionette lines: The deep creases that go from the corner of the mouth to the chin, and are a common part of the anatomy of any aging face. This expression is based on the lines created by the mechanical movement of the mouth of a marionette seen in puppet shows.

Medical aesthetician: A trained therapist working in a free-standing facility or in a plastic surgeon's office, who deals with skin care products and application of various technologies such as peels or microdermabrasion.

Mini facelift: A general term used when referring to an abbreviated facelift, also called a "short scar" facelift. Usually the neck, forehead, and eyelids are not done at the same time.

Nasolabial crease or fold: The junction of the fat of the cheek with the muscles around the mouth creates the nasolabial (nose to lip) crease or fold. With aging, the crease appears to get deeper as the cheek fat falls further down.

Ophthalmic plastic surgeon: Ophthalmologists who do general ophthalmology such as cataracts and eye disease frequently take extended training to become an ophthalmic plastic surgeon, and perform reconstructive and aesthetic surgery of the eyelids.

Orbit: The orbit refers to the part of the skull that houses the eye and has various components. For example, an orbital fracture is a fracture of one of the various bones that comprise the orbit.

Orbital fat: There are three fat compartments of the lower eyelid. Just the right amount of fat gives a smooth, youthful appearance. Too much fat can result in "bags" under the eyes. Orbital fat is also present under the upper eyelid.

Orbital septum: The septum is the thin cover of the orbital fat that is under the skin and muscle of the lower eyelid.

Orbicularis oculi: The muscle that encircles the orbit and helps form both the lower and upper eyelid. It is the muscle responsible for the crow's feet on the outside of the eyes when contracted.

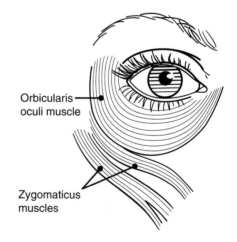

Otoplasty: An otoplasty is any operation dealing with the anatomy of the ears. It is a common operation for children with protruding ears.

Otolaryngologist: The technical term for an ENT or head and neck surgeon, a physician who traditionally deals with diseases of the ears, nose, and throat, including various forms of head and neck surgery.

Peel: A procedure that uses various types of acid solutions to minimize wrinkles and smooth the skin. Other methods that also remove the top layer of skin for the same purpose include laser treatments and dermabrasion.

Pixie ear: An expression meaning that the earlobe is pulled down following a facelift and is attached to the facial skin; its normal curvature is distorted.

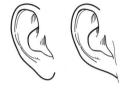

Normal earlobe   "Pixie ear"

Plastic Surgeon: By strict definition, this is a surgeon who has fulfilled the requirements necessary to be certified as a plastic surgeon by the American Board of Plastic Surgery.

Platysma: This is a rudimentary muscle of the neck, left over from the evolution of the human race. Its two front edges form the "cords" seen in the aging neck. It is the muscle still prominent in horses and other animals that is used for flicking off flies.

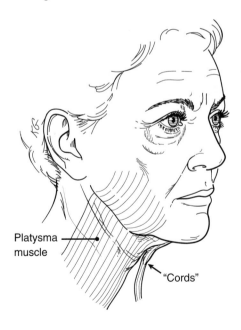

Platysma muscle

"Cords"

Positive vector orbit: An expression used to describe the anatomy where the lower eyelid glides gracefully down to the cheek, without the indention seen with patients with very hollow eyes or with excessive fat, which is seen with patients having a negative vector orbit.

Reconstructive surgeon: Reconstructive surgery refers to the surgical treatment by various specialties of deformities resulting from disease or trauma. There are many subspecialties, such as hand surgery or even gynecological surgery, which deal with reconstructive procedures.

Resurfacing: This term broadly refers to skin treatments that improve the appearance and texture of the skin, through the use of chemicals, lasers and light-based devices, or mechanical means such as dermabrasion.

Rhinoplasty: The operation used to make various types of changes to the shape of the nose.

Rhytidectomy: Rhytidectomy is the medical term for a facelift. "Rhytids" are wrinkles and "ectomy" means to cut out.

Scleral show: The sclera is the white portion of the eyeball; scleral show means that the lower eyelid is pulled down and too much white shows below the pupil. This

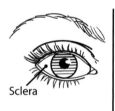

Sclera

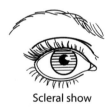

Scleral show

is a situation that may be normal, but also may occur after surgery.

Septal reset: An operation where the septum orbitale covering the fat of the lower eyelid is repositioned over the orbital bone. Its normal position is just within the orbit. This technique is used to rejuvenate the lower eyelid.

Septum (septum orbitale, orbital septum): The covering of the lower eyelid fat, underneath the muscle of the lower eyelid.

Sequela (plural = sequelae): Anything that may occur following an event. This is normally used to describe complications following surgery.

Short scar facelift: Facelifts that are normally done with an incision just in front of the ears, without an incision behind the ear.

Skin lift: A facial operation that deals only with lifting the skin of the face, also the oldest type of facelift procedure.

SMAS: An abbreviation for the "superficial musculo aponeurotic system," the muscle of the lower face (platysma) and its covering, first described in the medical literature in 1976.

Stigma of surgery (plural: stigmata): Refers to the characteristic signs of surgery, which are frequently unattractive.

Superior-medial (or superiomedial): This is a direction that is both upward and toward the middle of the face. The superior medial facelift moves the cheek tissue toward the eye and slightly toward the nose as well.

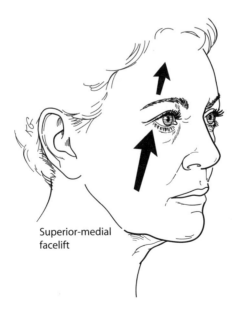

Superior-medial
facelift

Thread lift: A facelift technique attempting to lift the face with only barbed sutures placed down through the tissues. It has largely been abandoned.

Tragus: The cartilage tissue that is right in front of the hole in the ear. Many surgeons prefer that the facelift incision be made behind the tragus.

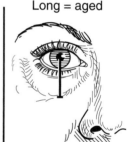

Tragus →

Ultrasound: A form of vibrating technology that is used for liposuction techniques, as well as other procedures.

Vectors: Directions used to describe the direction of lift in plastic surgery.

Vertical height of lower lid: The distance from the pupil to the border of the lower eyelid as measured in photographs. A short vertical height is normally seen in young patients, and the vertical height increases as the patient ages.

VERTICAL HEIGHT OF LOWER LID
Short = youthful | Long = aged

Zygomaticus: Muscles that start from the cheekbone and insert near the nose and corner of the mouth. There is a zygomaticus major and a zygomaticus minor.

Zygorbicular: A contraction of the word zygomaticus and orbicularis, used to describe a unique cheek lift technique that can be done with or without a Composite Facelift.

REFERENCES

Lemmon, M.L. & Hamra, S.T., Skoog Rhytidectomy: A Five-Year Experience. Plastic and Reconstructive Surgery 65:3, 1980.

Hamra, S.T., The Deep Plane Rhytidectomy. Plastic and Reconstructive Surgery 86:53, 1990.

Hamra, S.T., Composite Rhytidectomy. Plastic and Reconstructive Surgery 90:1, 1992.

Hamra, S.T., Composite Rhytidectomy. St. Louis: Quality Medical Publishing, 1993.

Hamra, S.T., Repositioning the Orbicularis Oculi Muscle in the Composite Rhytidectomy. Plastic and Reconstructive Surgery 90:14, 1992.

Hamra, S.T., Arcus Marginalis Release and Orbital Fat Preservation in Midface Rejuvenation. Plastic and Reconstructive Surgery 96:354, 1995.

Hamra, S.T., The Role of Orbital Fat Preservation in Facial Aesthetic Surgery: A New Concept. Clinics in Plastic Surgery 23:17. 1996.

Hamra, S.T., The Zygorbicular Dissection in Composite Rhytidectomy: n Ideal Midface Plane. Plastic and Reconstructive Surgery 102:5, 1998.

Hamra, S.T., Periorbital Rejuvenation in Composite Rhytidectomy. Operative Techniques in Plastic and Reconstructive Surgery, Vol 5, No 2 (May) 1998: pp 155-162.

Hamra, S.T., Frequent Facelift Sequelae: Hollow Eyes and the Lateral Sweep: Cause and Repair. Plastic and Reconstructive Surgery 102:5, 1998.

Hamra, S.T., Prevention and Correction of the "Face-lifted" Appearance. Facial Plastic Surgery 16:3, 2000.

Hamra, S.T., The Role of the Septal Reset in Creating a Youthful Eye-Cheek Complex in Facial Rejuvenation. Plastic and Reconstructive Surgery 113:2124, 2004.

INDEX

Index